From the book...

Wildflower Viewing (page 79)

Abbotts Lagoon is another exceptional wildflower spot, where brilliant swaths of goldfields and numerous other species cover the hillsides. Baby blue eyes, poppies, and more paint the bluffs behind Kehoe Beach, and the Coast, Bayview, and Tomales Point trails all provide excellent wildflower displays.

Bear Valley Trail to Divide Meadow and Arch Rock (Trip 1)

Look for newts crossing the moist trail in the rainy season, and winter wrens darting amid dense tangles of vegetation. Bracken, five-finger, and sword ferns coat the slopes. The heart-shaped leaves of wild ginger grow on the stream bank, and in spring, buttercups, milkmaids, and forget-me-nots sprout along the trail.

Coastal View Loop on the Bayview, Laguna, and Fire Lane trails (Trip 9)

The trail climbs moderately through open terrain, at first on a wide grassy path, narrowing and steepening as it reaches the crest of a low hill and a junction with the Fire Lane Trail. From this spot, you have views of the sweeping coastline of Drakes Bay, all the way to the point of Chimney Rock.

Point Reyes Beach (page 156)

Only sparsely covered by vegetation, the dunes often reach far inland, blown across the grasslands by the wind. The Great Beach itself stretches 11 miles along the Pacific Coast, exposed to high winds from the northwest and crashing surf with a strong undertow. The long and wild strand is perfect for an exhilarating walk, run, or romp with the dog.

Valley to Ridge Loop on Greenpicker, Ridge, Bolema, Olema Valley trails (Trip 26)

You may find the Ridge Trail muddy in the spring, with elderberry and huckleberry bushes spilling onto its course. It is a delightful trail nevertheless, and worth enduring these small bothers. Sunlight wafts through the trees, splaying on the forest's varied palate of green.

Bolinas Ridge Trail (Trip 35)

Especially popular with mountain bikers, the trail crosses rolling coastal rangeland, enters towering redwoods, and breaks into open chaparral before it reaches its southern trailhead at Alpine Road on Mt. Tamalpais. You'll enjoy far-reaching views of Bolinas Lagoon, Tomales Bay, and the Pacific Ocean.

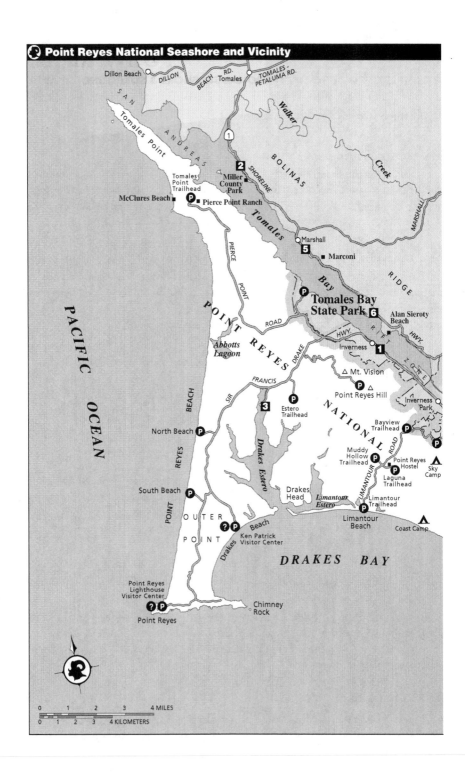

Point Reyes National Seashore and Vicinity

Dillon Beach

DILLON BEACH RD.
Tomales
TOMALES-PETALUMA RD.

SAN ANDREAS

Tomales Point

Walker

BOLINAS

Creek

MARSHALL

1

2

SHORELINE

Tomales

Miller County Park

Tomales Point Trailhead

McClures Beach ■

P Pierce Point Ranch

PIERCE

POINT

Marshall

5

■ Marconi

Bay

RIDGE

P Tomales Bay State Park 6

Alan Sieroty Beach

POINT REYES

ROAD

HWY.

Abbotts Lagoon

Inverness

△ Mt. Vision

PACIFIC OCEAN

FRANCIS

DRAKE

P △
Point Reyes Hill

Inverness Park

SIR

3

P Estero Trailhead

NATIONAL

Bayview Trailhead P

BEACH

North Beach P

Drakes Estero

Muddy Hollow Trailhead P

P Point Reyes Hostel

Sky Camp ▲

ROAD

Laguna Trailhead

REYES

South Beach P

Drakes Head

Limantour Estero

Limantour Trailhead P

LIMANTOUR

P Limantour Trailhead

POINT

OUTER POINT

Beach

?P

Ken Patrick Visitor Center

Limantour Beach

Coast Camp ▲

Drakes

DRAKES BAY

Point Reyes Lighthouse Visitor Center

?P

Chimney Rock

Point Reyes

N

0   1   2   3   4 MILES
0 1 2 3 4 KILOMETERS

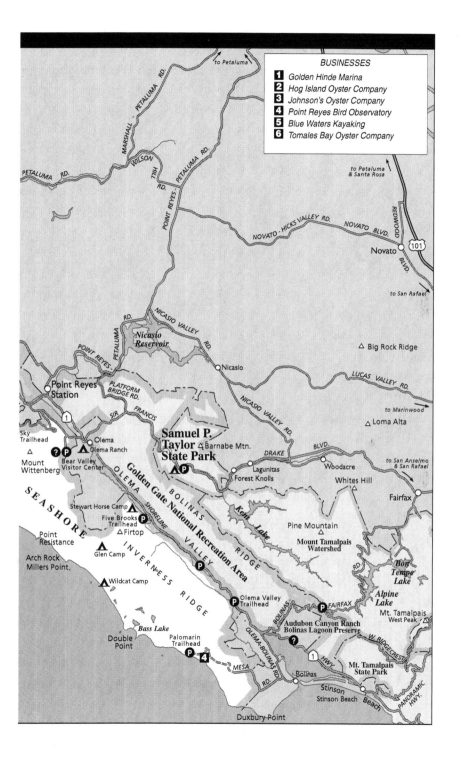

BUSINESSES

1. Golden Hinde Marina
2. Hog Island Oyster Company
3. Johnson's Oyster Company
4. Point Reyes Bird Observatory
5. Blue Waters Kayaking
6. Tomales Bay Oyster Company

to Petaluma

MARSHALL-PETALUMA RD.

WILSON RD.

7TH RD.

POINT REYES - PETALUMA RD.

PETALUMA RD.

to Petaluma
& Santa Rosa

NOVATO - HICKS VALLEY RD.

NOVATO BLVD.

REDWOOD BLVD.

101

Novato

to San Rafael

NICASIO VALLEY RD.

POINT REYES - PETALUMA RD.

Nicasio
Reservoir

△ Big Rock Ridge

LUCAS VALLEY RD.

Nicasio

NICASIO VALLEY RD.

to Marinwood

△ Loma Alta

Point Reyes
Station

PLATFORM
BRIDGE RD.

SIR FRANCIS

1

Sky
Trailhead

△
Mount
Wittenberg

Olema

Olema Ranch

Bear Valley
Visitor Center

**Samuel P.
Taylor
State Park**

△ Barnabe Mtn.

DRAKE

BLVD.

Lagunitas

Forest Knolls

Woodacre

Whites Hill

to San Anselmo
& San Rafael

Fairfax

S E A S H O R E

OLEMA

Golden Gate National Recreation Area

B O L I N A S

Stewart Horse Camp

Five Brooks
Trailhead

△ Firtop

Point
Resistance

Glen Camp

Arch Rock
Millers Point.

Wildcat Camp

I N V E R N E S S   R I D G E

SHORELINE

V A L L E Y

R I D G E

Kent
Lake

Pine Mountain
△

Mount Tamalpais
Watershed

Bon
Tempe
Lake

Alpine
Lake

Mt. Tamalpais
West Peak △

Bass Lake

Double
Point

Palomarin
Trailhead

4

Olema Valley
Trailhead

OLEMA-BOLINAS RD.

BOLINAS

FAIRFAX

Audubon Canyon Ranch
Bolinas Lagoon Preserve

1

HWY.

Mt. Tamalpais
State Park

W. RIDGECREST

MESA

RD.

Bolinas

Stinson
Stinson Beach   Beach

PANORAMIC HWY.

Duxbury Point

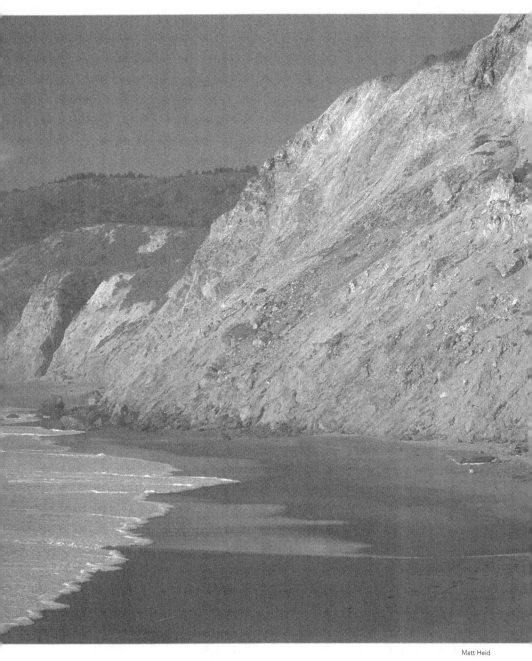

Matt Heid

The beach near Alamere Falls

POINT REYES

THE COMPLETE GUIDE TO THE NATIONAL SEASHORE & SURROUNDING AREA

JESSICA LAGE

WILDERNESS PRESS ... *on the trail since 1967*

BERKELEY, CA

Point Reyes: The Complete Guide to the National Seashore & Surrounding Area

1st EDITION 2004
  2nd printing 2006

Copyright © 2004 by Jessica Lage

Front cover photo copyright © 2004 by RichardBlair.com
Back cover photo copyright © 2004 by Jessica Lage
Interior photos, except where noted, by Jessica Lage
Maps: Ben Pease, Pease Press
Cover design: Larry B. Van Dyke
Book design: Courtnay Perry

ISBN 978-0-89997-350-0

Manufactured in the United States of America
Distributed by Publishers Group West

Published by: **Wilderness Press**
                1345 8th Street
                Berkeley, CA 94710
                (800) 443-7227; FAX (510) 558-1696
                info@wildernesspress.com
                www.wildernesspress.com

Visit our website for a complete listing of our books and for ordering information.

Cover photos: Cows, cliffs, and Drakes Bay from George Nunes' farm *(front)*;
                Abbotts Lagoon with wildflowers *(back)*

SAFETY NOTICE: Although Wilderness Press and the author have made every attempt to ensure that the information in this book is accurate at press time, they are not responsible for any loss, damage, injury, or inconvenience that may occur to anyone while using this book. You are responsible for your own safety and health. The fact that a trail is described in this book does not mean that it will be safe for you. Be aware that trail conditions can change from day to day. Always check local conditions and know your own limitations.

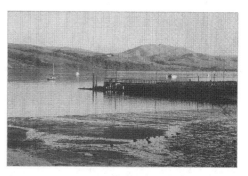

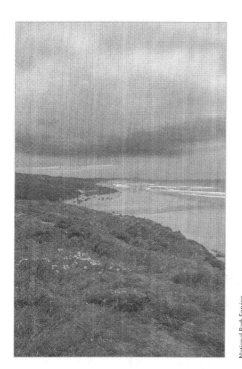

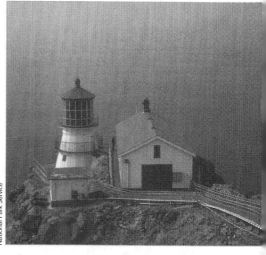

National Park Service

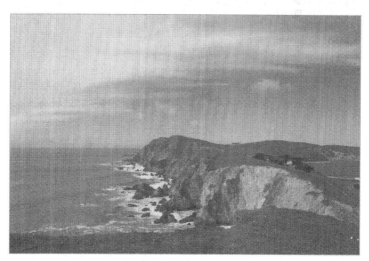

Top left: Wildflowers at Kehoe Beach. Top right: Pier on Tomales Bay.
Middle: Point Reyes Lighthouse. Bottom: Coast and bay view at Chimney Rock

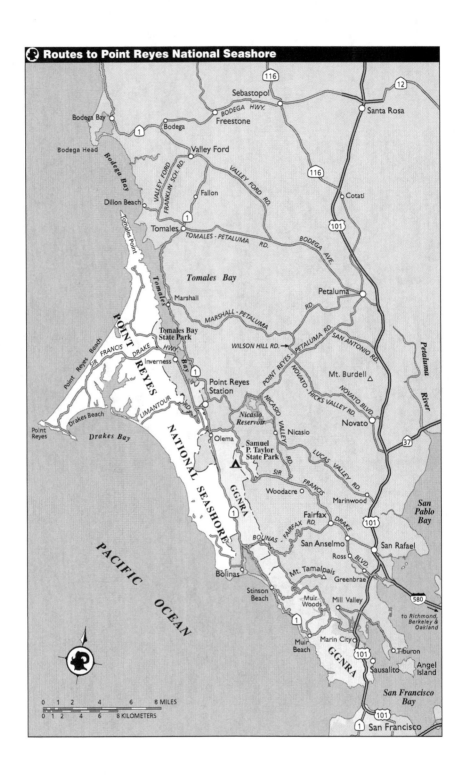

Routes to Point Reyes National Seashore

Contents

ACKNOWLEDGMENTS

Over the course of this project, I spoke with many people at Point Reyes National Seashore, all of whom were extremely helpful and informative. Thanks to John Dell'Osso, Chief of Interpretation, for meeting with me and for reviewing the manuscript. Bill Shook, Gordon White, Brannon Ketcham, Jane Rodgers, Shelly Benson, Ben Peterson, Kim Cooper, Sarah Allen, and Jennifer Chapman shared their extensive knowledge of Point Reyes with me and reviewed various parts of the manuscript. Many thanks to Carola DeRooy for her kindness in tracking down and scanning photos from the NPS archive. Gary Knoblock, Executive Director of the Point Reyes National Seashore Association offered encouragement and advice.

Point Reyes experts Dewey Livingston and Jules Evens read sections of the manuscript and provided helpful feedback. Gene Buvelot, Tribal Council member of the Federated Indians of Graton Rancheria, kindly spoke with me.

On several visits to her studio, Susan Hall was generous with her time and knowledge and always a pleasure to talk with. Lynn Giacomini Stray, Bob Giacomini, and Sue Conley made time in their busy schedules for several conversations with me.

Thanks to Jannie Dresser for encouraging the initial stages of the book and to Roslyn Bullas for shepherding it through to the end, with management and careful editing. Thanks also to Tom Winnett's keen eye. Ben Pease created the maps and was, as always, a pleasure to work with and a vigilant editor himself. Thanks to Jessica Benner for careful work on the maps and photographs, to Larry Van Dyke for the cover design, and Courtnay Perry for the interior design.

Enthusiasm, support, and accompaniment from my friends and family were indispensable. Jordan Lage provided entertainment on the trails as well as photos. Ray Lage, Ann Lage, and Katie Lage were crucial sources of encouragement. Ann and Katie also filled multiple roles as advisors, editors, proofreaders, and photographers, but above all as delightful companions who share a deep love for Point Reyes.

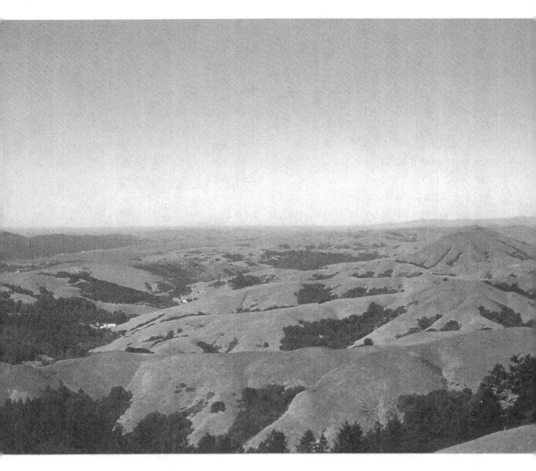

Tomales Bay and Black Mountain from Barnabe Mountain

Opposite page: Coastal swale at Abbotts Lagoon

Making the Most of Your Point Reyes Experience

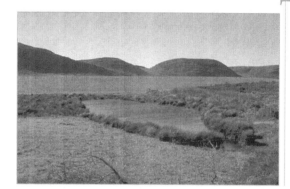

Chapter 1

POINT REYES: A PLACE APART

Just 30 miles from urban San Francisco, city routines fall away, the slow rhythm of rural life emerges, and the primordial cycles of the natural world reign on rocky shorelines and in tidal marshlands and bishop-pine groves. Little-traveled trails wander through Douglas-fir forests, beaches rim the coastline, whales swim in offshore waters, and wildflowers swathe coastal grasslands. In an hour's drive or less, across bridge, on highway and on winding country road, you can reach this place apart—Point Reyes.

An "island in time," Point Reyes has long been recognized as unique—distinct in character from its urban environs, unparalleled in ecologic diversity, and quite literally separated from the rest of Marin County and the Bay Area by the San Andreas fault. Point Reyes National Seashore encompasses 71,000 acres on the Point Reyes peninsula and draws 2.5 million annual visitors from around the world who explore the seashore's trails and beaches and visit nearby parks and preserves—Audubon Canyon Ranch, Tomales Bay and Samuel P. Taylor state parks, and the Golden Gate National Recreation Area. In small towns, visitors find gourmet food, comfortable accommodations, and scenic beauty—all the makings of a peaceful rural getaway.

Human settlement, exploration, exploitation, and recreation have left few places on Earth unaltered. While Point Reyes is a sanctuary of striking beauty and powerful natural forces, humans have "managed" the land and shaped the natural ecosystem for thousands of years. Coast Miwok, the area's first inhabitants, burned grasslands and undergrowth around oak trees and depended on the wealth of animal and plant life for food. In the 19th century, ranchers arrived on the peninsula, introducing new species of plants and animals and extinguishing others. As they developed what became the most productive dairy industry in California, ranchers constructed roads for travel, dammed streams, and built levees in marshlands. Later, weekenders and recreationists built homes and towns.

Knowing the human history of the land teaches us about the natural history. Letters from early visitors tell of animals now absent from the peninsula: a guest at one of the early ranches witnessed a duel between a bear and a bull—when grizzly bears still populated the area—and commented on the elk horns and bones scattered over the peninsula as the tule elk were hunted nearly to extinction.

Today, small communities, ranches, and national seashore lands exist side-by-side with this rich history. In the national seashore, the melding of agricultural land and wilderness area offers a offers a unique present-day experience. In a 22,000-acre ranching district in the northern region, 13 ranches still run beef and dairy cattle operations. And in an adjacent 32,000-acre wilderness area, the largest in any national seashore, you can wander old ranch roads that have been converted into trails and follow a route to the site of a once-planned

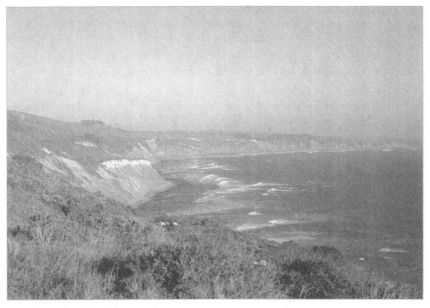

Coast Trail

subdivision; you can birdwatch on a tranquil estero, once a wharf busy with schooners ferrying between ranches and San Francisco markets; and you can look for wildflowers and tule elk on the site of a once-thriving dairy ranch. It is a wilderness shaped by humans, but where human intervention is now limited mostly to recreationists who travel the trails and camp at former ranch sites. The Point Reyes wilderness protects a remarkably diverse ecosystem—within the seashore live nearly 15 percent of California's plant species and nearly 30 percent of the world's marine mammal species. Close to 45 percent of all the bird species in North America visit the seashore.

A lot goes on behind the scenes at Point Reyes, both within and around the national seashore. Park biologists restore native plants to beachside dunes and administer birth control to a burgeoning population of tule elk. The National Park Service works with nearby communities to reduce fire risk. A local land trust partners with ranchers and farmers to preserve agricultural land around the national seashore. All of these activities affect your visit to Point Reyes, although you may not see them happening or even know they exist.

This book digs beneath the surface of Point Reyes and unearths its many layers, enriching your experience on the trails and beaches and in the bays and towns of the Point Reyes area. The beauty and complexity of each aspect of Point Reyes invite you in—to absorb the fantastic and exhilarating scope of the natural world, to drink in the uniqueness of each minute piece of nature, and to unwind in a quiet rural retreat.

USING THIS BOOK

Point Reyes: The Complete Guide to the National Seashore & Surrounding Area covers the entire Point Reyes area—the national seashore, Tomales Bay and Samuel P. Taylor state parks, Audubon Canyon Ranch Bolinas Lagoon Preserve, and activities and towns in the vicinity. The first chapter introduces you to the Point Reyes area with brief and vital information about how to spend your time here in every season of the year. Are you a first-time visitor? Find out where to go and what to see. Do you have only an afternoon in the park? Find out the best short hikes and activities. Do you have an entire day and want a challenging hike? You'll find that here too. Are you looking for a beach where you can take your dog? Do you want a great hike for a foggy day? A trail with spectacular wildflowers, top spots to see spawning salmon, the best hikes for kids. . . You'll find a suggested activity for any day in any season in Chapter 1.

Chapters 2 and 3 relate the natural and human history of the area. They will help you understand what you're seeing on the peninsula and help you appreciate and enjoy it.

Chapter 4 tells about the activities you can do in and around the national seashore, from hiking and kayaking to whale-watching and wildflower-viewing.

A tour of the area takes you from town to town, with details on what you'll find in each—galleries, bookstores, eateries, and fun events—and en route. You'll learn about food produced on local ranches and farms and—most importantly—find out where to sample their products.

Chapter 5 explores Point Reyes National Seashore itself, dividing the seashore into six main areas, some with multiple trails from one trailhead, such as Bear Valley and Five Brooks, and others with many trailheads, such as Limantour Road and Sir Francis Drake Highway. A brief introduction to each area and trailhead gives driving directions, facilities, and regulations.

The trips from each trailhead follow. An icon in the margin tells you if the trip is open to bikes and horses in addition to hikers. Each trip begins with an overview that summarizes the highlights, terrain, and trails, and tells you what to look for. If the trip sounds good, read on. Next, **Distance** is given in miles, calculated using the National Park Service map and other published maps and guides. (There are always discrepancies between distances given in books and maps and on park signs.) **Type** describes the route as loop, out-and-back, or shuttle. **Difficulty** rates the hikes from easy to strenuous, based primarily on distance and grade. **Facilities** tells where to find toilets, water, phone, and picnic tables; often there are no facilities at the trailhead or along the route. **Regulations** gives rules for dogs, bikes, and horses on the route. And finally, the **Description** takes you on the trip, describing the terrain, vegetation, and views, with detailed directions and mileages at certain points. Information in boxes and margins expands on what you'll see along the way—or sometimes on things you won't see, but that shape the landscape and your experience all the same.

Chapter 6 explores other parks and preserves in the Point Reyes area—Tomales Bay and Samuel P. Taylor state parks, Golden Gate National Recreation Area, and Audubon Canyon Ranch Bolinas Lagoon Preserve. Hikes and activities in each follow the same format as those in the national seashore.

MAPS

The two locator maps at the beginning of the book orient you to the area with geographic landmarks and towns, and display sites mentioned throughout the book. Eight trail maps correspond to trailheads and parklands in the surrounding area. Use these maps in conjunction with the trail descriptions in order to plan your trips. Trails are coded to show hiking, biking, and horse routes. Symbol marks campgrounds, picnic areas, parking, toilets, water, phones, wheelchair-accessible routes, shuttle stops, and ranches.

Map Legend

SYMBOLS

▲ Campground

⊕ Picnic Area

Ⓟ Trailhead Parking

Ⓡ Restroom

Ⓦ Drinking Water

Ⓒ Telephone

Ⓓ Disabilities Access Trail

Ⓢ Shuttle Stop (seasonal)

● Ranches

■▦ Buildings

BOUNDARIES

National Park and Recreation Area Boundary

State and Local Park Boundary

Overlap with Adjacent Maps

Vision Fire Area

ROADS

Paved highway

Secondary road

Unpaved road

Shuttle Route (seasonal)

TRAILS

Hiking, Equestrian and Bicycle Trail

Hiking & Equestrian Trail

Hiking Trail

Paved Bike Path

Other Trails (abandoned, not maintained, or not confirmed)

NATURAL FEATURES

Year-round Stream

Seasonal Stream

Body of Water

Spring

1407′ Elevation (feet)

△ Peak or Summit

Contours: 80 feet

Index Contours: 200 feet Datum is Mean Sea Level

KEY TO MAP COVERAGE

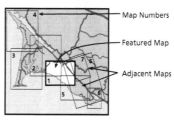

Map Numbers

Featured Map

Adjacent Maps

MAP NOTES:

Maps created from USGS 7.5° quadrangles:
Drakes Bay, Inverness, Tomales Point, Double Point, Bolinas, and San Geronimo.

Trails adapted from existing USGS data and National Seashore maps.
Selected trails field checked and remapped by Ben Pease, 2003.

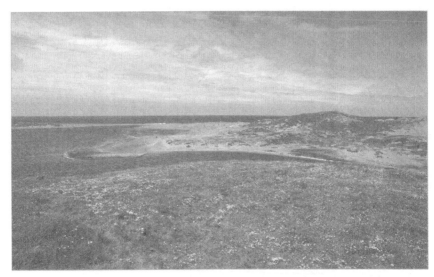

Wildflowers at Abbotts Lagoon, with the coast beyond

SEASONAL GUIDE

Seasons at Point Reyes can fool you. On a 70-degree day in January, you may wonder if you're south of the equator; and when you're shivering on a foggy July day, you might ask the same question. Clear days abound in fall and winter, spring ushers in changeable weather and strong breezes, and summer often brings dense coastal fog. Come to Point Reyes prepared for anything—fleece in August and shorts in December, rain jacket in April and T-shirt in November—but most of all, come prepared to be surprised and amazed at the beauty and variability of Point Reyes.

How do you decide what do to and when? The following are a few suggestions:

MONTH-BY-MONTH AT POINT REYES

January–February

Spring begins in winter at Point Reyes. Currant bushes bloom in coastal scrub, hound's-tongue and milkmaids decorate the forest, and occasional early-blooming Douglas iris peeks through grasses along coastal trails. January is the peak of the southern gray whale migration. Visit the lighthouse and Chimney Rock for the best whale-watching points; hikes along the Coast and Tomales Point trails and beach walks also may provide glimpses of passing whales. Look for winter birds at Limantour Spit, Drakes Estero and Abbotts Lagoon. Moderate inland temperatures make Bolinas Ridge and Olema Valley hikes pleasant.

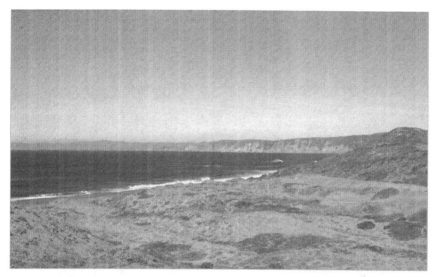
Dunes at Limantour Beach

March–April

By March, wildflowers begin unfurling in the green grasslands and beneath lush forest cover, building to brilliant April displays all over the peninsula. The short walks at Chimney Rock, Abbotts Lagoon, and Kehoe Beach are among the best for wildflowers. Hikes along the Coast, Fire Lane, and Laguna trails will take you through masses of blossoming ceanothus; in the Bayview/Muddy Hollow area, and on the Tomales Point and Estero trails, you'll find numerous species of wildflowers. Forested hikes from Bear Valley and Five Brooks display infinite shades of green and a more subtle wildflower show.

Whales and their young return north from Baja California in March and April; watch for them from the lighthouse and Chimney Rock, on the Coast and Tomales Point trails, and on beach walks along Limantour and the Great Beach. Hikes at Drakes Estero and Limantour Spit offer good views of harbor seals during pupping season (March through June), but bring your binoculars so you can get a good look without disturbing the animals. Hikes near the esteros are also good places to watch for spring-migrating birds.

Billowing white clouds in a bright blue sky characterize March and April's variable weather. Hot days intersperse weeks of chill and rain. Come prepared for strong winds at the headlands and on the beaches.

May–June

Most of May is still peak wildflower season at Point Reyes. (See the previously recommended trails for wildflowers.) As spring moves into summer, the days

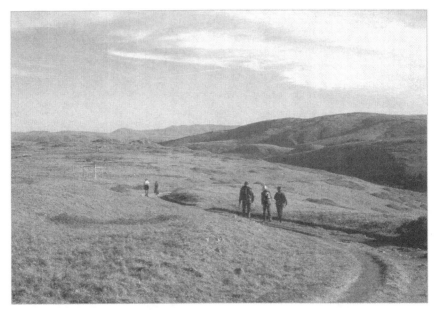
Hikers on Tomales Point Trail

lengthen, temperatures increase, and foggy days become more frequent. Come June, many wildflowers hang on in coastal scrublands and on beachside cliffs. Look for orange sticky monkeyflower on hikes to the coast from the Sky Trail—Laguna, Fire Lane, and Woodward Valley trails—and take the short walks to Kehoe and McClures beaches to see cliffside lizard tail and other beach plants.

July–August
Explore the trails in Tomales Bay State Park, where Inverness Ridge often keeps the fog from reaching these bayside beaches, and warmer water invites swimmers and waders. The grassy hills and redwood forests of inland Samuel P. Taylor State Park are also usually fog-free. The Bolinas Ridge Trail often bathes in sun when fog envelops the coast, as does the Olema Valley Trail. For a different experience, hike to the coast from the Sky or Bear Valley Trailhead to marvel at the puddles that collect from fog drip along the ridgetop trails and to see bright displays of sticky monkeyflower.

September–October
During the hot post-summer months, hikes in the wooded and riparian areas around the Bear Valley and Five Brooks trailheads provide shade and a chance to enjoy changing fall colors. Brilliant red poison oak leaves and more subtle shades of big-leaf maple, alder, and willow enliven the forest. Leafless buckeyes reveal graceful branches, and berries hang from honeysuckle, huckleberry, and elderberry

bushes. Since September and October are usually the hottest months of the year, you might want to avoid the exposed trails that head to the coast from the Sky and Bayview trailheads. From Palomarin, the hike along the open bluffs of the Coast Trail may be hot, but Bass Lake is a cool and refreshing reward.

The fall bird migration is at its height in September and October, and the short trails along Abbotts Lagoon, Kehoe Marsh, Limantour Spit, and Olema Marsh are good places to observe it.

November–December
The peninsula's first storms often arrive in November, clearing the air and bringing great coastal views. By December, traces of green appear in the grasslands and rain moistens the forests, nurturing new growth, luscious ferns, and delicate mosses. You'll have superb views from the Tomales Point, Coast, and Sky trails.

Shorter days begin to limit your hiking time as winter nears, but take advantage of the earlier sunsets and plan to be out as the sun falls below the horizon. Panoramic views from the Inverness Ridge Trail make it a great place to see the peninsula bathed in brilliant shades of pink—reflected in Drakes and Limantour esteros—and still make it back to a trailhead with enough light to see your route.

CULTURAL AND NATURAL HISTORY EVENTS
Month-by-month, here are the cultural and natural history events happening in Point Reyes National Seashore.

January
Pacific gray whale migration
Elephant seals breeding
Coho salmon spawning
Shorebirds and waterfowl
Anniversary of naming of Point Reyes (January 6, 1603)

February
Pacific gray whale migration
Elephant seal breeding
Steelhead trout spawning

March
Wildflowers in bloom
Heron and egret nesting at Audubon Canyon Ranch
Harbor seal pupping
Pacific gray whale migration
Elephant seal breeding

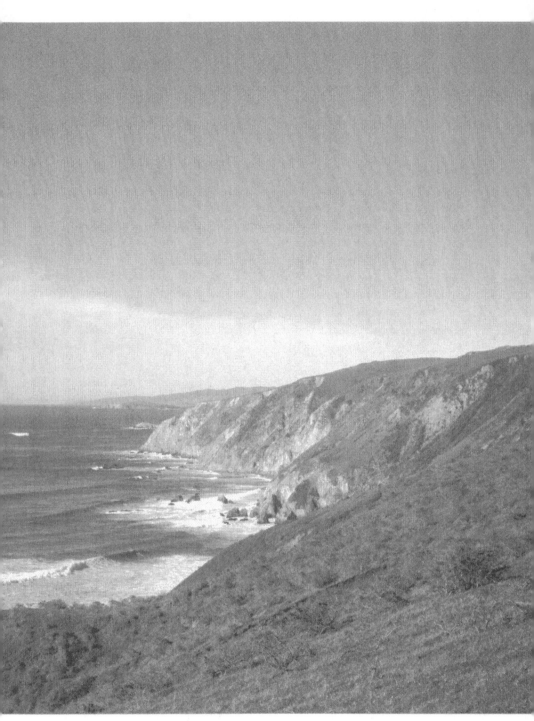

The coast along Tomales Point

April
Native American Spring Festival at Kule Loklo
Wildflowers in bloom
Heron and egret nesting at Audubon Canyon Ranch
Harbor seal pupping
Pacific gray whale migration
Elephant seal breeding

May
Ranches and Rolling Hills landscape art show (Marin Agricultural Land Trust)
Evening lighthouse programs
Wildflowers in bloom
Heron and egret nesting at Audubon Canyon Ranch
Harbor seal pupping

June
Heron and egret chicks at Audubon Canyon Ranch
Wildflowers in bloom
Harbor seal pupping
Evening lighthouse programs

July
Native American Big Time Festival at Kule Loklo
Heron and egret chicks at Audubon Canyon Ranch
Point Reyes Open Studios
Evening lighthouse programs

August
Tule elk rut
Shorebirds and waterfowl
Evening lighthouse programs

September
Tule elk rut
Shorebirds and waterfowl
Evening lighthouse programs
Park anniversary (September 13, 1962)

October
Harvest Moon
Harvest Festival at the Farm (MALT)
Tule elk rut
Shorebirds and waterfowl
Evening lighthouse programs

November
Elephant seal breeding
Point Reyes Open Studios
Shorebirds and waterfowl

December
Pacific gray whale migration
Elephant seal breeding
Shorebirds and waterfowl
Lighthouse birthday (1870)
Coho salmon spawning

ACTIVITIES AND HIKES
BY THEME AND WEATHER

SUGGESTIONS FOR FIRST-TIME VISITORS
Mt. Vision Drive for a view of the peninsula (Trip 17)
Interpretive walks at Bear Valley for an overview of the park's cultural, natural, and historical and geological significance (see page 101)
Lighthouse and Chimney Rock (especially in spring for whales and wildflowers; see pages 160, 157)
Historic dairy ranch at Pierce Point (see page 174)
Bear Valley Visitor Center (see page 101)

WHAT TO DO IF YOU HAVE ONLY AN AFTERNOON
Tried and true suggestions
Hike to Divide Meadow (Trip 1)
Interpretive walks at Bear Valley (see page 101)
Mt. Vision Drive (Trip 17)
Beach walk at Limantour (Trips 15 and 16)

Off-the-beaten-track suggestions
Marshall Beach (Trip 21)
Shell Beach, Tomales Bay State Park (see page 209)
Oyster tasting (see pages 91)

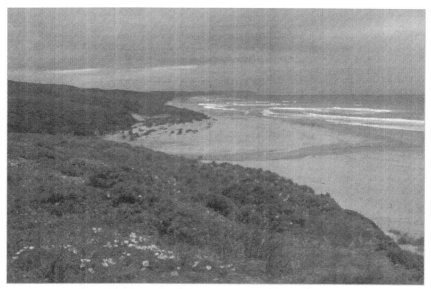

Wildflowers at Kehoe Beach

PICNICS

Limantour and Drakes beaches (on Drakes Bay)
Pierce Point Ranch (at an historic dairy ranch)
Tomales Bay State Park (Hearts Desire and Alan Sieroty Beach on Tomales Bay)
Samuel P. Taylor (among creekside redwoods)

GROUP GATHERINGS

Hearts Desire Beach and picnic area (Tomales Bay State Park)
Bear Valley headquarters

WILDFLOWER TRAILS

Chimney Rock Trail (Trip 20)
Abbotts Lagoon Trail (Trip 22)
Tomales Point Trail (Trip 24)
Marshall Beach Trail (Trip 21)
Coast Trail just south of Arch Rock (Trips 1, 5, 30)

CREEK AND WATERFALL TRAILS

Coast Trail to Alamere Falls (Trip 31)
Bear Valley Trail (Trip 1)
Olema Valley Trail (Trips 26, 36)
Rift Zone Trail (Trip 6)
Stairstep Falls, Samuel P. Taylor State Park (Trip 40)

VIEWS TRAILS
Estero Trail to Drakes Head (Trip 18)
Coast Trail (Trips 4, 5, 31)
Chimney Rock Trail (Trip 20)
Tomales Point Trail (Trip 24)
Inverness Ridge Trail (Trip 12)
Woodward Valley Trail (Trips 4, 8)
Barnabe Mountain, Samuel P. Taylor State Park (Trip 41)

BIRDING TRAILS
Bayview Trail (Trips 11, 12)
Estero Trail (Trip 18)
Chimney Rock Trail (Trip 20)
Abbotts Lagoon Trail (Trip 22)
Bear Valley Trail (Trips 1, 3, 4, 5, 30)

FOGGY DAY TRAILS
To revel in the fog: Sky Trail along Inverness Ridge (Trips 3, 4, 8)
    Tomales Point Trail (Trip 24)
To escape the fog: Olema Valley Trail, Rift Zone Trail (Trips 6, 36)
    Bolinas Ridge Trail, Golden Gate National Recreation Area (Trips 35, 36)
    Tomales Bay and Samuel P. Taylor state parks (Trips 33, 34, 38–41)

HIKES TO THE COAST
From Bear Valley Trailhead (Trips 1, 3, 4)
From Sky Trailhead (Trips 8, 10)
From Point Reyes hostel (Trip 14)
From Five Brooks (Trips 27, 28, 30)
From Palomarin (Trip 31)

ACTIVITIES FOR/WITH KIDS
Interpretive Trails: Kule Loklo, Earthquake Trail, Woodpecker Trail, Nature
    Trail to Indian Beach (Tomales Bay State Park), Pioneer Nature Trail (Samuel
    P. Taylor State Park)
Beaches: Hearts Desire (Tomales Bay State Park), Limantour, Drakes
Backpack Trips: Coast Camp

HISTORIC SITES
Upper Pierce Point Ranch
Radio Corporation of America (RCA) facility (on Sir Francis Drake Highway)
Point Reyes lighthouse
Lifeboat Station

WHEELCHAIR-ACCESSIBLE
Audubon Canyon Ranch picnic area, bookstore, and display hall
Abbotts Lagoon Trail, first 0.4 mile (Trip 22)
Estero Trail, first 0.5 mile (Trip 18)
Earthquake Trail
Lighthouse Visitor Center
Bear Valley Visitor Center
Drakes Beach Visitor Center

BEACHES YOU CAN DRIVE TO
Point Reyes Beach North and South
Drakes Beach
Hearts Desire Beach (Tomales Bay State Park)

BEACHES ACCESSIBLE BY A SHORT WALK
Indian Beach, Tomales Bay State Park, 0.5 mile
Pebble Beach, Tomales Bay State Park, 0.5 mile
Shell Beach, Tomales Bay State Park, 0.3 mile
Kehoe Beach, 0.6 mile
Limantour Beach, 0.2 mile
McClures Beach, 0.4 mile
Palomarin Beach, 1 mile
Point Reyes Beach at Abbotts Lagoon, 1.2 miles
Marshall Beach, 1.2 miles

BEACHES YOU CAN HIKE TO
Wildcat Beach
Kelham Beach
Secret Beach
Sculptured Beach
Santa Maria Beach

BEACHES WHERE YOU CAN TAKE YOUR DOG
Note: Dogs must be on a 6-foot leash and may be restricted during snowy plover nesting season
Kehoe Beach
Point Reyes Beach
Limantour Beach (southern end)

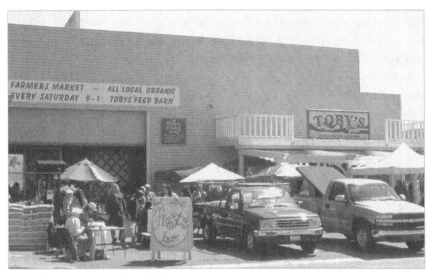
Farmers' market, Point Reyes Station

OVERNIGHTS
Hike-in: Wildcat Camp, Coast Camp, Glen Camp, Sky Camp
Drive-to: Samuel P. Taylor State Park
Boat-in: Tomales Bay beaches
Bike to: Coast Camp, Wildcat Camp
In the redwoods: Samuel P. Taylor State Park
On the coast: Wildcat Camp, Coast Camp
On the ridge: Glen Camp, Sky Camp
Great for kids: Coast Camp

FAIRS AND FESTIVALS
Farmers' market: Saturdays in summer from 9 A.M. to 1 P.M., Toby's Feed Barn, Point Reyes Station
Western Weekend and 4-H parade (Point Reyes Station): June
Point Reyes Open Studios: July 4th weekend and Thanksgiving weekend
Harvest Festival at the Farm (Marin Agricultural Land Trust): October
Ranches and Rolling Hills **landscape art show** (MALT): May
Strawberry Festival at Kule Loklo: April
Big Time Festival at Kule Loklo: July

Opposite page: View across Tomales Bay from Marshall Beach

Natural History

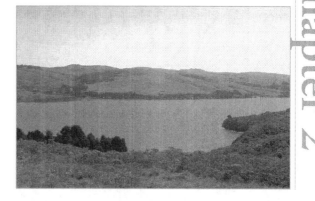

Chapter 2

On April 18, 1906, the infamous San Francisco earthquake ruptured the ground, cutting a crack from Bolinas Lagoon to Tomales Bay. The land on either side of the fault wrenched horizontally a full 16 feet near the town of Point Reyes Station! (Reports cite 20 feet near Tomales and 18 feet at the Point Reyes lighthouse.) The earthquake revealed the power and dynamism of this complex fault zone, and geologists quickly realized that the earth had been moving slowly but substantially along the San Andreas fault for millions of years. The fault separates the Pacific Plate from the North American Plate—and the Point Reyes peninsula from the mainland. Often called an island because of its geologic history, the peninsula is also an island of natural history—an outpost where a distinct geology and a mosaic of habitats have created a unique ecosystem and a remarkable experience for visitors.

For a more complete look at this area's fascinating natural history, see Jules Evens' exceptional book, *A Natural History of the Point Reyes Peninsula*.

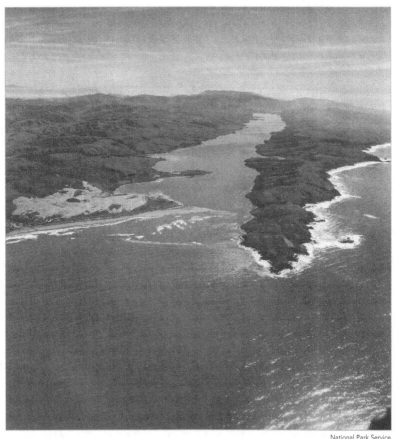

Aerial view of Tomales Point and Tomales Bay

TOPOGRAPHY

Understanding the topography of Point Reyes will help you unravel the complexity of the peninsula: by knowing the lay of the land, you'll be able to decide where you want to spend your time. Within just 100 square miles, the Point Reyes peninsula displays a huge variety of land forms and environments.

To enter the unique world of Point Reyes, visitors must first cross the San Andreas fault, the thread by which the peninsula hangs from the mainland. The long trace of the fault runs beneath Tomales Bay, meets land at the bay's southern tip, and continues south through Olema Valley to Bolinas Lagoon, where it reenters the ocean. Pastoral Olema Valley is a showcase for the out-of-the-ordinary topography that fault zones often exhibit: small freshwater lakes (sag ponds) in unlikely places (on the crest or slope of a hill), creeks with complex drainage patterns, and uplifted and folded hills and ridges.

Inverness Ridge runs southeast-northwest along the peninsula. On the Tomales Point Trail, you are on the northern reaches of the ridge, where it rises gently from the west shore of Tomales Bay. To the south, the ridge slopes upward, first to Mt. Vision and then higher to Point Reyes Hill (the second highest point on the ridge and a great spot to take in the panorama of the area). A few miles south, Mt. Wittenberg crowns Inverness Ridge at 1407 feet; its slopes descend to Bear Valley, the only breech in the ridgeline and a nearly level route to the coast.

At its southern end, Inverness Ridge eases into Bolinas Mesa, a level, wave-cut marine terrace northwest of Stinson Beach. On the Coast Trail, you'll be hiking on the coastal plateau that extends from Bolinas Mesa to Limantour Estero, a prominent feature of this coastline. Just south of Bear Valley, fault action and erosion caused a large landslide (nearly 5 miles long and at least a mile wide) that covers the once-continuous terrace and forces the trail up the ridge, along steep cliffs that drop to the ocean. Offshore, sea stacks and arches reveal the erosive power of the ocean. North of Bear Valley, the slopes of Inverness Ridge descend more gradually to the coast, and you can continue on the level terrace toward Limantour Beach.

On your way to the lighthouse and Chimney Rock, you'll pass Drakes Estero, which, like Limantour Estero, was a valley that filled with water eons ago when the coast was submerged. At the westernmost tip of the peninsula—Point Reyes itself—the lighthouse stands on rocky headlands above the ocean, and high cliffs drop precipitously to the water. Stretching northward from the point, Point Reyes Beach (the Great Beach) extends for 11 miles, and its high sand dunes often blow inland across pasturelands of the outer point. Beyond the Great Beach, Tomales Point extends high above the ocean to the mouth of Tomales Bay, where Inverness Ridge culminates in rocky granitic headlands.

GEOLOGY

The 1906 earthquake revealed the most significant structural feature of the Point Reyes peninsula: the San Andreas fault zone. Were it not for the fault, this little triangle of land, nearly 30 miles long and 12 miles wide, would have a vastly different history, and indeed would not be in its present location 30 miles north of San Francisco.

Geologists believe that the Point Reyes peninsula was once farther south—adjacent to the Monterey Bay area, about 60 million to 15 million years ago. Over the subsequent millennia, the peninsula has crawled northward at an average rate of about 2 inches per year. Some of this movement is what geologists call "creep"—slow, intermittent movement we can't detect. However, most of the journey occurs in leaps and bounds, as when the peninsula moved by as much as 20 feet in 1906.

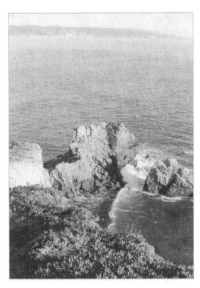

Chimney Rock

Evidence for the peninsula's movement north is in the rocks: the geology east and the geology west of the fault reveal a dramatically different histories. The peninsula's granitic bedrock identifies it as part of a massive granitic block (the Salinian Block) that extends west of the San Andreas fault from Bodega Bay south to the Monterey peninsula. Similarities in the composition of the granite in the Monterey-area Santa Lucia Mountains and on the Point Reyes peninsula suggest a common origin. Franciscan rocks—chert, serpentine, graywacke, and conglomerate—found on the Marin mainland do not exist west of the San Andreas fault.

The peninsula's granitic foundation is its oldest rock. Exposed on the rocky cliffs above the ocean at Tomales Point and near the lighthouse, the hard granite is highly resistant to batterings by the Pacific's waves. Younger rocks and marine sediments overlay the granite on most of the peninsula. Point Reyes Conglomerate, a unique composition of hard sedimentary rock, is the oldest of these marine sediments and occurs only in one spot on the peninsula—at Point Reyes itself. Look for a fascinating outcropping just above the stairs to the lighthouse: embedded egg-size pebbles of volcanic rock and several blocks of granite and chert give the conglomerate a warty appearance. Similarities between the volcanic rocks in the conglomerate and those found at Point Lobos in Monterey are further evidence that the Point Reyes peninsula was once attached near Monterey.

Along the spine of Inverness Ridge from Tomales Point to Mt. Wittenberg, only a thick layer of soil and vegetation covers the peninsula's granitic rocks. The marine sediments—Monterey shale and Laird sandstone—which once covered this northern section of Inverness Ridge, have eroded away over time. They still overlay the granite on Inverness Ridge south of Mt. Wittenberg to Bolinas Mesa, and extend over the western slopes to the coast. A soft, light-colored muddy sediment originally called the Drakes Bay Formation but now referred to as the Purisma Formation covers the cliffs and hillsides around Drakes Bay. Its fine sand contains abundant fossils of invertebrates and other marine animals like seals, fish, and whales. The cliffs at Drakes Beach—likely those that reminded Drake of the white cliffs of Dover—reveal this formation most dramatically.

Visit the Earthquake Trail at the Bear Valley Visitor Center to see the crack in the earth from the 1906 quake first-hand and to learn more about the earthquake.

The 1906 Earthquake—The Human Story
Most people have heard stories about San Francisco after the 1906 earthquake and subsequent fires, but few know that the quake was centered near Point

Reyes and that the greatest displacement along the fault—some 20 feet—occurred along Tomales Bay. At 5:13 A.M. on April 18, 1906, in the town of Point Reyes Station, the 5:15 train to Sausalito tipped over from the force of the quake as it was preparing to leave the station. The log-cabin post office in Inverness caved in, bathhouses on the beach fell over, and summer homes slid off their foundations. The east side of Tomales Bay received

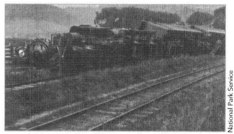

Derailed train in Point Reyes Station, 1906

National Park Service

the brunt of the damage, especially the railroad tracks and trestles along the shore. The quake demolished the church in Tomales, and the hotel at Marshall slid into the bay.

CLIMATE

Climate not only influences how we spend our day at the seashore, but it shapes every part of what we see when we visit—from the whales we spot offshore to the cattle grazing on the headlands. It is a vital element of the ecosystem. Were it not for Point Reyes' particular climate, its natural and human histories would be quite different: the cold, nutrient-rich upwelling in the Pacific supports the abundant marine life that inhabits the waters off the coast—the whales, seals, and sea lions that we scan the waters for and observe along the shoreline. The thick fogs that sweep over land provide moisture for a long growing season and foster the area's prime pastureland.

A typical Mediterranean climate—warm, dry summers and cool, rainy winters —characterizes Point Reyes. Moderated by the ocean, temperatures at Point Reyes are remarkably uniform throughout the year: midsummer and midwinter averages differ only by about 10 degrees. However, within the park, numerous microclimates create vastly different environments; in a single day, and within only a few miles, you may encounter great variations in temperature, rainfall, wind, and fog.

> *"There was a driving wind from the sea. The whole country round about was enveloped in a fog so dense that the eye could not penetrate it more than a dozen rods."*
> —Oscar Shafter, in a letter to his father, 1858

> *"All who have tried to explore the Point Reyes dunes and downs in the midst of a cold summer fog can fully sympathize with the early English visitors and even forgive them the slight exaggerations that color their record."*
> —Thomas Howell, *Marin Flora*

Early visitors to Point Reyes frequently commented with great discouragement on the heavy fogs that blanketed the headlands and beaches. During the spring and summer, the upwelling along the Pacific Coast brings cold water to the ocean's surface; fog then forms when offshore air cooled over the water meets warm inland air swept to the coast by winds. The dense mists contribute

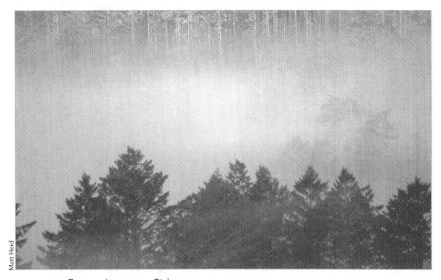

Matt Heid

Fog on Inverness Ridge

significant moisture to the vegetation—as much as 10 inches of precipitation per year. Thick summer fogs on Inverness Ridge drench the tall grasses and create muddy puddles in the trail, reminiscent of winter rain.

Discouraging as this may sound to the visitor seeking sunny weather, microclimates at Point Reyes often come to the rescue. Even in summer, when fogs are most common and thickest, you are likely to find blue sky and sun, especially east of Inverness Ridge. The ridge often shelters the eastern slopes, the inland valleys, and Tomales Bay beaches from fog and wind. Interior and coastal temperatures may differ by as much as 20 degrees, especially in summer, when fog is most likely on the headlands.

Rainfall on the peninsula also varies greatly between inland and coastal microclimates. Most precipitation falls on the peninsula between November and March. In inland valleys like Bear Valley, the average rainfall is about 36 inches a year, far heavier than the 12- to 19-inch average that falls on the outer headlands at the lighthouse.

Although strongest in spring, wind is usually a year-round presence on the headlands and the Pacific beaches. The annual maximum averages 43 miles per hour, but rare southerly windstorms in November and December bring the strongest blasts: the highest recorded wind velocity is 130 mph at the Coast Guard Station near the lighthouse. Winds usually pick up in the afternoon, so try to plan your trip to the lighthouse or Chimney Rock for the morning. Afternoon winds also make boating on Tomales Bay and the esteros more enjoyable in the morning.

PLANT COMMUNITIES

An astounding range of plant communities exist within just 100 square miles at Point Reyes. At 38 degrees latitude, Point Reyes is a convergence point for plants typical of coastal areas to the north and those to the south; it lies near the southern tip of the Douglas-fir range and the north edge of the coastal scrub community. Oak trees, bishop-pine forests, grasslands, marshes, and intertidal areas all thrive in the multiple microclimates that the peninsula's complex topography and distinct soil types create. Point Reyes National Seashore is home to 900 species of flowering plants (including 15 percent of all the species that grow in California) and 50 rare plant species.

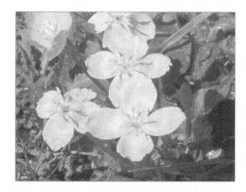

Suncups

BISHOP-PINE FOREST

"Never far from the ocean, their striking bluff-top groves seem designed by Japanese printmakers."

—Elna Bakker

The bishop-pine forest at Point Reyes is one of the most extensive in California, although a large part of it burned in the 1995 Vision Fire. Once widespread along the California coast and into Baja California, bishop pines (*Pinus muricata*) now grow only in scattered stands, always within a few miles of the ocean. The pines often take on a bonsai-like shape, contorted by strong winds and dwarfed by thin, nutrient-poor soils. Under ideal conditions—plenty of fog and precipitation and acidic soils with high moisture content—bishop pines grow into tall, regal trees, reaching heights between 40 and 70 feet.

Bishop pines belong to a family of "closed-cone" pine trees—a thick, resinous coating seals their cones. Rather than opening at maturity, the cones require fire (or in rare cases, a particularly hot day) to open and release their seeds. Without the cycle of periodic fires that release the seeds and generate new growth, the forest will die out after about 100 years or less. Bishop pines in a single stand tend to be the same age, because all the trees usually have resprouted after the most recent fire.

At Point Reyes, bishop pines grow almost exclusively on granitic soil, thus restricting the forest to the northern half of Inverness Ridge. Since the 1995 Vision Fire, the pines have sprouted all the way down the coastal slope, although these young trees may not have the right conditions to evolve into a mature forest. Around Sky Camp on Inverness Ridge, the bishop-pine forest gradually gives way to the Douglas-fir forest prominent on the southern ridge.

Where soil conditions allow, other trees join the bishop-pine forest. In moist and shady areas, California wax myrtle, coffeeberry, huckleberry, and salal grow under dense tree cover. Ceanothus, manzanita, and madrone take advantage of the exposed spaces between trees in drier forests. Bay laurel trees grow in damp canyons, with tanbark oak and Douglas-

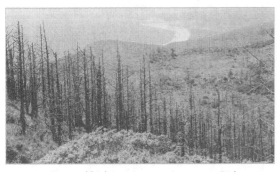

Burned bishop pines on Inverness Ridge

The gray-green needles of bishop pines are short and stiff, about 3 to 6 inches long, and grow in clusters of two. The cones have a distinctive whorled pattern and are about 2½ to 3 inches long. Bishop pines usually have a dense, rounded crown, and few lateral branches.

fir on arid slopes above. The Vision Fire burned much of the mature bishop-pine forest in Point Reyes National Seashore, so the best place to see the established stands is in Tomales Bay State Park, which escaped the fire.

DOUGLAS-FIR FOREST

"The Douglas-fir is a grand tree; some individuals within the Seashore rival redwoods in girth and height."

—Jules Evens

Not a fir at all, the misnamed Douglas-fir (*Pseudotsuga menziesii*) has a prominent presence on the Point Reyes peninsula. The towering trees (some measure between 300 and 400 feet in height) grow on the southern end of Inverness Ridge, in the deep shale and sandstone that overlie the granite base rock. The Douglas-fir forest at Point Reyes is an outpost of the dense and uniform forests that grow to the north, as close as Sonoma County and throughout western Oregon and Washington, although it is missing several companion tree species that grow in the northern forests.

Douglas-fir has short, soft, dark-green needles that grow all the way around the twigs. The cones hang from the tips of the twigs, 2½ to 4 inches long, with distinctive bracts between the scales. The bark of young trees is smooth and greenish-gray; as the trees mature, the bark becomes dark brown, thick, and furrowed.

At Point Reyes, bay laurel trees join the Douglas-fir forest, and poison oak climbs tall trunks. In riparian areas around Bear Valley (near Coast, Olema, and Bear Valley creeks), the forest is dense and the understory lush. Ferns and wild ginger thrive in the moist soils, and long trains of lichen hang from tree branches. The forest along the crest of Inverness Ridge and the slopes south of the Five Brooks Trailhead are drier, with a brushier understory of tanbark oak, huckleberry, coffeeberry, and honeysuckle.

NORTHERN COASTAL SCRUB

Downslope of the Douglas-fir ridgeline, a rich mosaic of coastal scrub emerges on the western flanks of Inverness Ridge and stretches to shoreline bluffs. From afar, coastal scrub appears to be a uniform cover of shrubby vegetation, but up-close you will find an astounding array of color, texture, shape, size, and fragrance. The deep, intoxicating aroma contained in oils and resins on leaves is one of coastal scrub's most delightful characteristics.

Coastal scrub covers slopes and canyons along the Pacific Coast from Baja California to southern Oregon. Plants from grassland, chaparral, forest, coastal bluffs, and interior hills and canyons often find a place in this diverse community. In southern and northern California, coastal scrub takes on identifiably different associations. At Point Reyes, the southern community tapers off, after a long transition zone from San Luis Obispo County to Marin County. Some typical southern species, such as California sagebrush, grow only as far north as Point Reyes, where plants in the northern scrub community begin to replace them.

On the western, scrub-covered slopes of Inverness Ridge, coyote bush (*Baccharis pilularis*) and bush lupine (*Lupinus arboreus*) are most prominent. On shady, relatively moist north-facing hillsides, fronds of bracken and sword fern, tangles of blackberry, low-growing salal, tall cow parsnip, and graceful currant bushes also thrive. South-facing slopes nurture plants that grow in drier, sunnier locations, such as sticky monkeyflower, California sagebrush, yerba buena, and coffeeberry. Since the Vision Fire, ceanothus is perhaps the most prominent shrub on coastal slopes at Point Reyes; poison oak is ubiquitous, growing in tall, dense thickets or low bushes.

ERADICATING EXOTIC PLANTS

Exotic plants aren't the purview of only expert gardeners. Even in areas where we may expect to see only a natural environment—in national parks like Point Reyes, for example—the native vegetation shares its terrain with plants from all over the world. We are constantly reminded that for all its natural beauty, Point Reyes is not a pristine ecosystem, but rather one that has been heavily managed throughout its human history.

The nonnative plants that grow on the peninsula today arrived here at different points throughout history, both accidentally and intentionally. Some of the earliest invasives on the peninsula were European annual grasses. Their seeds first arrived in the early 1800s, on the hooves of Californio's longhorn cattle. Later, dairy ranchers planted Italian rye grass and cultivated hay, oats, and barley for feed. Early ranchers also planted another common nonnative—the blue gum eucalyptus tree. These eucalyptuses, used as windbreaks around ranches, are a poster-tree for invasive species. Like European grasses and other exotic plants, eucalyptuses grow and spread rapidly, taking over large swaths of land. They and other nonnatives become invasive because the diseases, parasites, and animals that kept them in check in their original homes are not present in their new habitat.

Point Reyes National Seashore is home to over 900 species of flowering plants, including 46 species designated as rare. Of these, about 300 are nonnative species—one-third of the seashore's entire plant population. Botanists are concerned about these exotic plants not because they "don't belong" here, but because they interfere with the complex web of relationships between native plants and animals that underlies a healthy ecosystem. Invasive species are the second major cause of extinction (after habitat destruction) of rare plants.

The National Park Service has taken on several projects in the seashore to eradicate invasive species, aiming to increase biodiversity and protect rare

Coastal scrub plants sometimes also appear in the sandy soils of the outer point. A small-leaved, low-growing variety (var. *pilularis*) of coyote bush predominates here, joined by yellow-flowering bush lupine and lanky grasses.

NORTHERN COASTAL PRAIRIE AND COASTAL RANGELAND

Large tufts of native grasses once flourished on the Point Reyes mesa, thriving in the long coastal growing season. Buttercups, blue dicks, and ferns sprouted in small pockets of bare soil between grass clumps. When agriculture took hold on the peninsula, the coastal prairie largely disappeared, as European annual grasses— arriving on the hooves or coats of animals and in feed supplies—gradually took

species. One project you might see is underway at the lighthouse: expansive mats of ice plant (*Mesembryanthemum*, a native of South Africa) on the rocky cliffs here consumed the habitat of some rare plants, including coast rock cress (*Arabis blepharophylla*), north coast phacelia (*Phacelia insularis* var. *continentis*), and Point Reyes rein orchid (*Piperia elegans* spp. *decurtata*). (Point Reyes is the only place in the world this rein orchid grows.) As you walk from the parking area to the lighthouse, you'll see large clumps of weeded ice plant. This exotic is fairly easy to pull up, but the thick, fleshy leaves are extremely heavy, so removing the weeded plants is not feasible.

Since ice plant resprouts very little, it makes a satisfying target for a restoration project: plots in the lighthouse project began with 89 percent ice-plant cover; since they were weeded, only 1 percent has grown back—an unusual success rate in a removal project. Another invasive plant project aims to eradicate ice plant and European dunegrass from the dunes at Abbotts Lagoon. (See page 31.)

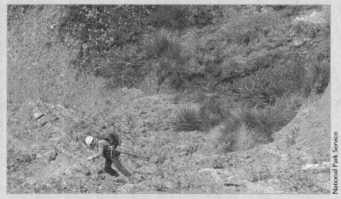

The NPS hires climbers to rappel down the lighthouse cliff face and pull invasive plants over the natives. Damaged by intense cattle grazing, the slow-growing perennial grasses could not compete with the annuals.

Today, grazed rangeland covers most of the rolling grasslands on the outer point, although a few remnants of the pre-agriculture habitat prairie survive. Low wildflowers and grasses cover drier, level plains, and moisture-loving sedges and rushes flourish in wetter swales. Pacific hairgrass (*Deschampsia holiciformis*), a hearty bunchgrass, still grows on Point Reyes prairies, despite grazing pressure. Two species of native bentgrass, awned bentgrass (*Agrostis aristiglumis*) and Point Reyes bentgrass (*A. clivola* var. *puntareyensis*) survive only on the coastal prairies of Point Reyes.

Virtually the entire eastern edge of Tomales Bay is coastal prairie. Native grasses and plants persist, although they are increasingly affected by velvet grass and tall fescue. These two invasives take over native vegetation, turning the prairie into a monoculture.

Even among the dominant swath of annual grasses, wild bulbs like Douglas iris, blue dicks, blue-eyed grass, and lilies sprout in spring. California buttercup, lupine, checkerbloom, gold fields, baby blue eyes, and footsteps of spring also brighten the green fields with a tapestry of color. A rare variety of yellow meadow foam (*Limnanthes douglasii sulphurea*), found only in Point Reyes, bursts into flower in March and April in vernal pools and wet swales; rushes, sedges, and bracken ferns grow among the grasses.

In 1980, a botanist found the rare Sonoma spineflower (*Chorizanthe valida*) growing on grazed coastal rangeland in Point Reyes National Seashore. Once common in Marin and Sonoma counties, the flower was thought to be extinct until the Point Reyes population—the only one in the world—was discovered. In 2000, biologists and volunteers from the Point Reyes National Seashore Association, the National Park Service, and the California Native Plant Society planted the spineflower in four plots in the park, where it is slowly gaining ground.

Rare Plant-A-Thon

One weekend a year, groups of plant lovers head into the field to document the vast array of rare plants in Point Reyes National Seashore. In what is now an annual event, volunteers—many professional or amateur botanists—and experts from park staff and the California Native Plant Society help provide vital information about plants that grow in the park's forests, grasslands, and dunes. Park biologists use these reports in resource-management decisions that allow the park to continue to coexist as a recreation unit, a working agricultural area, and a unique and treasured piece of the larger ecosystem.

Often the Rare Plant-A-Thon turns up good news. New discoveries of rare plant species on the peninsula continue to surprise park biologists, as do new populations of previously documented species. In 2002, the surveyors discovered two species biologists didn't know existed on the peninsula: the endangered robust spineflower (*Chorizanthe robusta*) and the rare Humboldt Bay owls clover (*Castilleja ambigua ssp. humboldtiensis*). They found 21 unrecorded populations of rare plants within the park in 2001, and 23 populations in 2002. The Rare Plant-A-Thon is one part of the park's many ongoing projects that aim to recover rare species, help them flourish, and eventually remove them from the "rare" list. This event also demonstrates that volunteers can contribute significantly to the health of the park.

If you'd like to participate in the next Rare Plant-A-Thon, call park biologists at (415) 464-5100 for more information.

COASTAL CLIFFS AND DUNES

The granite coastal cliffs at Point Reyes are surprisingly resistant to the ocean's battering, yet like coastal dunes, they are not a particularly hospitable environment for plants. The few plants that survive in these harsh oceanside conditions have certain characteristics that help them counter the dehydrating effects of strong winds, salt air, and low precipitation: their succulent leaves store water and a ground-hugging growth pattern protects them from the elements. Plants that live on the cliffs seek out protected crevices, where they find some accumulation of soil and rainwater, and shelter from the wind. The only moderate condition in their environment is temperature, which provides a year-round growing season for coastal-strand plants, most of which are perennials.

Two fleshy-leaved, moisture-storing plants that peek from cliffside crannies are live-forever (*Dudleya*) and stonecrop (*Sedum*). The yellow-flowering lizard tail (*Eriophyllum staechadifolium*) is also common on Point Reyes cliffs. A non-native that has become almost ubiquitous on California's coastal bluffs is ice plant (*Mesembryanthemum*). Introduced from South Africa, ice plant invades bluffs and dunes, reducing plant diversity by discouraging native plants and increasing the salt content in the soil.

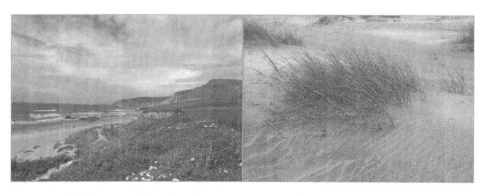

Wildflowers at Kehoe Beach   Dune grass

On coastal dunes at Point Reyes and northward along the California coast, beach grass predominates. The most common grass at Point Reyes, European beach grass (*Ammophila arenaria*), native to the Mediterranean, was first introduced on the Pacific Coast in Golden Gate Park in the 1890s as a dune stabilizer. The beach grass quickly overran the native American dune grass (*Elymus mollis*), limiting the growth of native plant species and restricting burrowing places for animals. The underground roots (rhizomes) of beach grass and American dune grass stabilize the dunes, creating a foredune that keeps the sand from advancing and shelters the plants just inland.

On the lower beach, beach grass, sand verbena, and sea rocket are among the few plants that live nearest the ocean. Behind the foredune, a greater variety of plants benefit from the protection the dunes provide. Dune lupine (*Lupinus chamissonis*)— low-growing and long-blooming, with fragrant flowers and silvery foliage—and coyote bush (often of a prostrate variety with small leaves) predominate. They are joined on the sandy mounds by trailing strands of beach morning glory (*Calystegia soldanella*) and sand verbena (*Ambronia umbellata*), coast buckwheat (*Eriogonum latifolium*), seaside daisy (*Erigeron glaucus*), and beach strawberry (*Fragaria chiloensis*).

MARSHLANDS

A great range of plants and animals make their home in marshlands, one of the most diverse habitats at Point Reyes. As human activities have altered traditional boundaries between salt, brackish, and freshwater areas, much of the marshland on the peninsula has been lost and flow patterns changed. Early ranchers and settlers restricted tidal influences with roads, culverts, and levees to create more pastureland. The levee road between Point Reyes Station and Inverness Park isolated what is today the freshwater Olema Marsh from what was once a brackish extension of Tomales Bay. In the 1940s, land at the southern end of Tomales Bay was turned into pastureland; the National Park Service recently acquired the land and is working to restore its marsh habitat.

The shores of Tomales Bay, Bolinas Lagoon, and Drakes and Limantour esteros comprise the peninsula's 1000 acres of salt marsh. Plants in the salt marshes are distributed according to how much saltwater exposure they can withstand. Pickleweed (*Salicornia virginica*) and saltgrass (*Distichlis spicata*) grow close to the coast, in water with a high saline content. Where freshwater gains influence, sea thrift (*Armeria maritima*), and alkali heath (*Frankenia*) appear.

In freshwater marshes, sedges, rushes, alder, and willows take over. Olema Marsh is the most extensive freshwater marsh at Point Reyes and one of the largest in Marin County. The upper reaches of Abbott's Lagoon, Drakes and Limantour esteros, and Kehoe Marsh also host freshwater species, including bog

The dunes of Point Reyes' Great Beach support a rich yet vulnerable ecosystem. This sandy environment is home to 11 federally listed endangered plant and animal species—including the snowy plover—all threatened by the spread of invasive plant species. (See page 170 to find out more about snowy plovers.) Dense mats of European dunegrass and ice plant crowd out native plants and reduce nesting and foraging area for animals. In an on-going habitat restoration project, the National Park Service is targeting a stretch of the Great Beach near Abbotts Lagoon—the most extensive native dune habitat in the park and a popular spot for birdwatchers, beachgoers, and wildflower-seekers.

Ecosystems are in constant flux, so when the subject of habitat restoration comes up, many people ask, "restoration to *what*?" Over the last couple of centuries, humans have planted exotic plants, introduced nonnative animals, logged forests, and dammed lakes, all intending to improve on nature. Too often, in doing so we have only damaged natural ecological processes. Restoration seeks to recover natural systems and the biodiversity they create, and to restore sustainable processes to the ecosystem.

For restoration projects at Point Reyes, the park carefully chooses the targeted sites. Areas with well-defined boundaries offer the best hopes of truly eradicating invasive species. In the relatively contained area around Abbotts Lagoon, the dune restoration project aims to establish an environment in which snowy plovers, endangered lupine, layia, and American dunegrass all coexist, unthreatened by the spread of European dunegrass and ice plant.

Restoration work itself is dirty and back-breaking: laborers dig several feet in the sand to reach the tough roots of grasses and ice plant. It is always a long-term proposition. Nevertheless, on the dunes behind the Great Beach, native plants have begun to take hold and spread over the sandy hillocks. Dune restoration at Abbotts Lagoon is one small but important step in Point Reyes National Seashore's efforts to recover healthy ecosystems and restore rare plants.

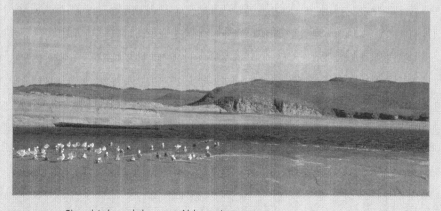

Shorebirds and dunes at Abbotts Lagoon

lupine (*Lupinus polyphyllus*), seep monkeyflower (*Mimulus guttatus*), and various rushes (*Juncus*).

INTERTIDAL COMMUNITY

The shoreline zone between the high and low water marks is called the intertidal community, habitat for an array of marine plants, from giant kelps to microscopic algae. What we call seaweeds are a type of green, brown, or red algae, although the color we see is not necessarily related to the algal classification. Algae are plants, but they lack true flowers, leaves, and roots, and reproduce with spores.

Where each type of algae grows within the intertidal zone is dictated by its amount of exposure to air—or how often the tide covers it. The plants in the splash zone—on rocky shores—tolerate prolonged periods without water; those that live in the lower and subtidal zones need less sunlight and are not disturbed by wave action.

Look for seaweeds along the beaches at Point Reyes, especially offshore of Sculptured and Kehoe beaches and near the mouths of Drakes and Limantour esteros.

ANIMALS

LAND ANIMALS

The Point Reyes grasslands, forests, and seashore once teemed with animals. Grizzly bears, mountain lions, and coyote roamed the hills, salmon and trout swam the bays and streams, and deer and tule elk grazed the prairie. The animals provided Coast Miwok with a rich food supply for thousands of years. Many of these species persist, and you will likely encounter them as you hike Point Reyes trails and walk its beaches. For nearly two centuries now, another species has grazed the peninsula's grasslands, also highly valued as a food source:

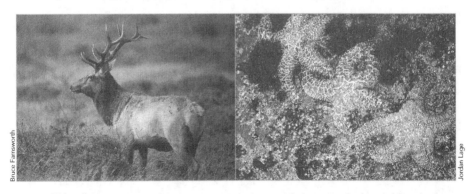

Tule elk   Sea stars at Sculptured Beach

cows. First longhorn and then dairy cattle were introduced to the peninsula, and today, both dairy and beef cattle remain.

The following is an overview of some of the land animals at Point Reyes. After a 100-year hiatus, the Park Service reintroduced **tule elk** to their native range at Point Reyes with great success. Three species of **deer** live on the peninsula: black-tailed or mule deer, native to the area, were hunted intensely a century ago, and today compete with tule elk for forage; fallow deer, native to the Mediterranean and Asia Minor, and axis deer, native to India, were both introduced to the peninsula in the mid-1900s. Some fallow deer are white in color, often an uncanny sight on Point Reyes hillsides.

Bobcats and **mountain lions** both rove the peninsula, preying on rodents and rabbits in the case of the smaller bobcat, while mountain lions, or cougars, eat deer, skunks, raccoons, and even bobcats. Visitors to the peninsula stand a good chance of seeing a bobcat, but rarely glimpse the more elusive mountain lion.

The small **gray fox** darts along trails and through low bushes and grasses. With its gray back and reddish legs, the gray fox is often mistaken for the **red fox**, a less-common resident of the peninsula. Fox feed mostly on rodents, insects, berries, and grasses. The **coyote**, once common at Point Reyes, now rarely visits the peninsula, although it frustrates sheep ranchers in West Marin by preying on their herds.

Small **cottontail or brush rabbits** frequently scamper across trails, seeking refuge in the dense cover of chaparral and coastal scrub. Resembling jackrabbits, **black-tailed hares** spring about on long and strong hind legs that allow them to move quickly and avoid predators.

Bears at Point Reyes

The grizzly bear, icon of Yellowstone and the interior West, once also roamed coastal California in abundance. The wealth of food sources at Point Reyes provided grizzly bears with a year-round feast of berries, nuts, and fish. In the 1800s, these predators became prey, as early settlers and gold miners shot grizzlies for sport and to protect livestock. The last grizzly in Marin County was shot in the 1880s.

Although black bears don't usually share grizzly habitat, preferring forest to the grizzly's open range, historical documents record a few sightings of black bears in wooded areas of the peninsula like Inverness Ridge. With the grizzly bear long extinct in California, more and more black bears have turned up near the coast. In 2003, a black bear was found rummaging in the trash at the Point Reyes hostel—the first in over a century to visit Point Reyes—and subsequently visited nearby areas. It remains to be seen whether this heralds the return of the species, or only a brief appearance.

AQUATIC ANIMALS

The cold-water upwelling that occurs off the California coast in spring and summer creates one of the most productive and diverse marine habitats in the entire world. A vast supply of small organisms like krill and algae flourish in the nutrient-rich water and draw mammals, fish, and seabirds. Within a relatively small area, a complete range of marine habitats thrive, from deep ocean to estuarine and intertidal, and support a remarkable variety of plants and animals. The largest concentration of breeding seabirds in the United States, 36 marine mammal species, and 20 percent of California's breeding population of harbor seals all depend on these waters.

Visitors to Point Reyes National Seashore experience this rich marine environment as they view the abundance of marine mammals and seabirds that pass by or stop over in the seashore—to feed, mate, or give birth—at some point during the year.

Sanctuaries for Sealife

The offshore waters around Point Reyes support some of the most diverse marine life in the world. They also sustain a number of commercial fisheries and some of the West Coast's heaviest shipping traffic. To protect the marine environment, in 1981 Congress designated 948 square miles off the coast as the Gulf of the Farallones National Marine Sanctuary, encompassing the waters from Stinson Beach to Bodega Bay, including the Farallon Islands, Tomales Bay, and Bolinas Lagoon. Sanctuary status precludes drilling and mineral exploration and other activities damaging to the health of the marine ecosystem, although it provides no protection against oil spills from tankers outside its boundaries.

About 20 miles offshore from the Point Reyes lighthouse, at the edge of the Continental Shelf, an underwater island called Cordell Bank sits on the tip of a long granite peninsula. Deep water surrounds the islands' peaks and valleys on three sides. Cordell Bank National Marine Sanctuary, established in 1989, protects the submerged island and 526 square miles around it.

After a close-call with extinction and a long absence from Point Reyes, **elephant seals** once again visit and breed on these beaches. The Elephant Seal Overlook and the Lifeboat Station at Chimney Rock, and the South Beach Overlook near the lighthouse are all good places to look for elephant seals from late November through early March. (See page 158 for more information about these intriguing animals.)

The largest concentration of **harbor seals** in California gathers along the Point Reyes shoreline and feeds in the offshore waters. You'll likely see their torpedo-shaped bodies on tidal flats near Drakes Estero, Limantour Spit, and Double Point. (See page 142 for more information about harbor seals.) **California sea**

lions breed, feed, and bark loudly on offshore rocks at Point Reyes, the northern tip of their breeding grounds. Sometimes confused with harbor seals, sea lions can be distinguished by their external ear flaps. They move about on land more easily than seals because they can rotate their pelvis and use their back flippers to propel themselves.

The most commonly sighted cetaceans at Point Reyes are **gray whales** on their annual migration between feeding grounds in Alaska and breeding sites in Baja. (See page 73 for more about gray whales and whale-watching.) **Blue** and **humpback whales** also travel along the coast, farther from land than gray whales. You're less likely to see them, but to picture their size, imagine three school buses lined up end-to-end. An average blue whale, the largest animal on earth, is about 70 to 90 feet long.

Several species of **dolphins** and **porpoises** live in the waters off Point Reyes; watch for their graceful arcing bodies as you scan the ocean for whales.

For more information about marine mammals, check out the interpretive programs at the lighthouse and visit the Elephant Seal Overlook at Chimney Rock. You can also contact the Gulf of the Farallones National Marine Sanctuary or the Marine Mammal Center at the Marin Headlands.

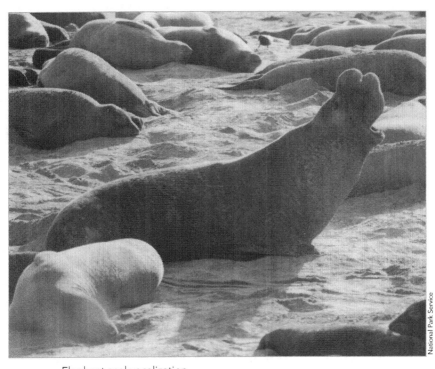

National Park Service

Elephant seal vocalization

COHO SALMON AND STEELHEAD TROUT
RESTORATION

When rains begin to fill West Marin creeks in early winter, you have a good chance of sighting coho salmon and steelhead trout on their way upstream to spawn, thanks to restoration projects at Point Reyes National Seashore and nearby watersheds. Until a few decades ago, West Marin creeks, like others up and down coastal California, teemed with coho salmon and steelhead trout. Grizzly bears feasted on the abundant fish, and Coast Miwok celebrated their arrival each winter. But the coho and steelhead population in West Marin has dropped dramatically since the 1940s, and statewide about 94 percent fewer fish swim in California's rivers, streams, and ocean. It's no mystery why the population has declined so much in the past several decades: most injurious have been the dams that block migratory paths, and the logging, construction, and poor agricultural practices that send sediment into streams. Less detrimental, but certainly not helpful, are overfishing and genetic intermixing with hatchery-raised fish, which weakens the survival abilities of wild coho and steelhead. Add the unpredictable natural fluctuations like floods, droughts, and ocean conditions to these human-driven impacts and you have two species that need quite a bit of help to regain a healthy habitat.

The National Park Service Restoration Program

At Point Reyes, the proximity of agricultural and national park lands often makes decisions about land use and practice difficult. When coho salmon and steelhead trout were listed as threatened species, the National Park Service designed a restoration program to research habitat conditions and monitor fish populations. The success of the program rests on collaboration between National Park Service scientists and staff, land owners, school groups, and volunteers. After several years of gathering data about fish numbers and learning about the streams, the program has instilled a deeper awareness and understanding of the riparian ecosystem, and has provided information that the park and its collaborators can put to use to improve the ecosystem, thus enhancing fish habitat.

Water level is key to the survival of salmon and steelhead fry (recently hatched fish) through the summer after their birth, but farms and ranches in the area also depend on water to nourish their crops. Fish and organic lettuce compete for water during the summer low-flow season. Meeting the needs of both agriculture and fish is one major challenge of the restoration program, especially in Pine Gulch Creek in Olema Valley. By working with the organic farmers who operate in the watershed, the program has successfully implemented innovative water-management practices that provide water for crops as well as salmon.

In addition to water flow, other elements of a healthy riparian ecosystem are gravel stream bottoms (fish survive better there than in streams with sandy bottoms) and plenty of leafy branches extending over the water (bugs drop from the leaves into the water and the waiting mouths of fish). Park staff and volunteers have planted willows along stream courses, helping to reduce erosion and sediment accumulation and providing foliage cover.

Life Cycle

Coho salmon are anadromous fish, spending most of their lives in the sea but returning to freshwater streams to give birth. They hatch in freshwater creeks and migrate to the ocean after about a year. Toward the end of their three-year life cycle, their powerful olfactory sense guides the salmon back to their natal watershed.

As they make their way upstream to spawn, females take on a bronze cast while male salmon turn dark red and develop an enlarged, hook-shaped upper jaw. Their bodies become tattered and scratched. Females lay their eggs in small depressions (redds) that they create in the gravel on the stream bottom. Males fight each other to establish dominance, and the victor fertilizes the eggs.

Salmon reproduce only once in their lifetime; they give up feeding during spawning and devote all their energy to reproduction. After salmon spawn, they die. Some live only 24 hours in freshwater; at most, they spawn 21 days after entering the stream. The new generation of fish hatched from the fertilized eggs will supply food for wildlife and humans; however, the death of the parent fish is perhaps an even more important contribution to the ecosystem. A vital step in the natural cycle, their death allows the survival of other plants and animals: the weakened salmon and their decomposing bodies provide food for animals and release nitrogen for plants. They nourish even their own offspring, which feed on the mayflies and other insects that lay their eggs on the carcasses of the parent fish.

For humans, the life cycle of coho salmon takes on a mythic quality. Their powerful sense of smell, their return to their natal watershed, and their self-sacrificing reproductive act fascinate us. In West Marin, this fascination has led to action. In addition to the National Park Service, several local citizen groups have started creek restoration projects in response to the decimation of coho and steelhead habitat over the past few decades. These groups lead walking tours to prime spawning spots where curious nature-lovers watch for the colorful fish making their way upstream.

Although their life cycle differs from that of coho, steelhead trout are also anadromous fish, migrating from freshwater river to ocean, and back to the river to give birth. Unlike coho, steelhead make several journeys upstream in their lifetime.

Where to See Salmon

Look for spawning coho salmon in West Marin creeks during December and January, especially a couple of days after a big rainstorm. The best spot to see salmon in Point Reyes National Seashore is **Olema Creek** at a roadside pullout along Highway 1 (mile marker 22.67). Park your car safely off the road while you look for salmon jumping or resting in the creek near the fish-passage structure, built as part of the park's restoration project.

Several sites in Samuel P. Taylor State Park offer good salmon viewing. See the section on that park for specifics.

Salmon-watching Tips

You're most likely to see salmon if they don't see you. Stay on the banks of the creek away from the water. Don't throw anything into the creek, and be sure your footing doesn't cause rocks or soil to slide into the water. Disturbing salmon habitat is harmful to the fish and reduces your chances of seeing salmon spawning and resting on reeds.

BIRDS

Over 490 bird species visit the Point Reyes peninsula each year, drawing human visitors from all over the world to behold their profusion and diversity. The varied habitats at Point Reyes attract a wide range of bird species that don't usually gather in one location. The temperate climate makes a good breeding and wintering spot for migrants. Rarities find their way to Point Reyes' coastal location with surprising frequency, so not only are you likely to see a great many birds here, but you stand a good chance of sighting birds not common to the Bay Area.

Each season brings a different grouping of birds to Point Reyes, according to annual cycles of food sources and migration and breeding patterns. The migratory seasons, traditionally fall and spring, extend almost year-round at Point Reyes as hummingbirds return from Mexico in February and Arctic birds arrive in August on an early start to their journey. But migration accelerates in fall and spring, and these months are the most active, as geese, loons, pelicans, warblers, and many more stop off on the peninsula. In summer, when the days are longest and food is abundant, Point Reyes is a breeding grounds for more than 100 species of birds. In winter, shorebirds and seabirds flock to the shorelines, mudflats, and bays of Point Reyes, and landbirds head to the forests to feast on berries and acorns. Raptors search for small rodents in grasslands and coastal scrub.

For the best birding spots in the Point Reyes area, and some of the birds you're likely to see on and around the peninsula, see pages 75–77.

THE POINT REYES BIRD OBSERVATORY

The Point Reyes Bird Observatory is a nonprofit membership-supported organization that studies birds and other wildlife and their ecosystems. Based at Palomarin in Point Reyes and the Farallon Islands, the observatory carries out projects throughout the western United States, monitoring and collecting data that help to protect birds and conserve habitats. PRBO was the first bird observatory in the United States (established in 1965), and its innovative programs and research have made it an international model.

At the PRBO Palomarin visitor center, you can learn more about bird habitats and watch research in action at banding demonstrations: join PRBO biologists on a short walk to collect birds from nets, and then watch the banding, weighing, and measuring process back in the lab. Demonstrations take place from sunrise until 12 P.M., Tuesday through Sunday from May 1 to Thanksgiving. Between Thanksgiving and April 30, demonstrations take place only on Wednesday, Saturday, and Sunday. You're most likely to see the birds between 8 A.M. and 11 A.M. Strong wind, heavy fog, and rain all close the nets. Call ahead to check conditions.

A self-guided nature trail makes a three-quarter-mile loop from the visitor center. PRBO experts lead a 2-hour bird walk the first weekend of each month to a nearby research area. Learn about fall migrants around Bolinas, snowy plovers at Abbotts Lagoon, shorebirds at Limantour Estero, and much more. Trips are free for members and $10 for non-members. Check the PRBO website for details.

Driving Directions: From Hwy. 1, at 4.5 miles north of Stinson Beach and 9 miles south of Olema, turn west at the often unsigned Bolinas turnoff. Continue 1.7 miles to Mesa Rd., and turn right. Follow Mesa Rd. for 2.7 miles and turn left into the Point Reyes Bird Observatory driveway.
Facilities: Restroom, water, phone, visitor center
Hours: Sunrise to 5 P.M., every day of the year
Contact: (415) 868-1221; www.prbo.org

THE VISION FIRE

On September 30, 1995, a group of boys made an illegal campfire in the bishop-pine forest on the western slope of Inverness Ridge. The boys extinguished the fire before they left, but its embers retained their heat and smoldered for several days. By the afternoon of October 3, a fire apparently had spread beneath thick duff to the roots of a nearby tree, and the tree burst into flames.

Initially, fire fighters successfully contained the fire to a small area, but strong, gusty winds quickly spread the burning embers to dense and flammable vegetation. Several spot fires began around the original fire, and hot weather, low humidity, and the high winds catapulted it into an intense firestorm. At its height, the fire reached up to 3000°F and consumed an acre every five seconds.

The fire swept through the bishop-pine forest on Inverness Ridge, jumping from one tree crown to the next, leaving virtually no tree untouched. It quickly reached a heavily vegetated residential neighborhood on the ridge where narrow, tree-lined roads made it difficult for firefighters to reach the homes and for residents to evacuate. Within the first 24 hours after the fire was reported, 45 homes had burned.

By the second day of the fire, it had swept over the ridge and down the coastal slope. The dense vegetation and thick debris that had accumulated on the forest floor over nearly a century without fire fueled the blaze, and winds of 40 to 50 miles per hour propelled the flames across firebreaks and over the coastal hillsides to the ocean. Then the winds changed direction, and the fire moved back up the slope, expanding to the north and south as it went. Firefighters had established firebreaks along several trails, and had hoped to stop the blaze at Limantour Road, but ultimately it was the natural barriers of the ocean and the esteros that were most effective in stopping the fire.

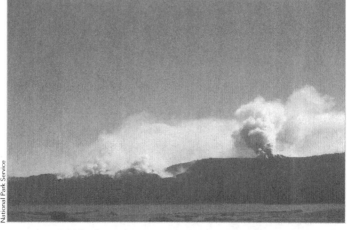

National Park Service

Smoke from the Vision Fire rising over Inverness Ridge

After firefighters declared the fire 100 percent contained on the evening of October 7, it flared up again, and they remained on the scene for another week. In the end, the fire had consumed 12,354 acres—15 percent of Point Reyes National Seashore—45 homes on Inverness Ridge, and three other structures. More than 2000 firefighters, nearly half of them inmates from correctional institutions, came from all over the state to fight the fire. Miraculously, not a single person was injured or killed in the fire or firefighting efforts. The fire cost $6.2 million for suppression, at least $50 million in property damage, and the costs of the post-fire restoration work have yet to be totaled.

FIRE AFTERMATH

Once the Vision Fire was contained, the story of the fire had only just begun. The aftermath of the fire—research on the effects of the fire on the park and on plants and animals, and changes in fire management—continues today, years after the fire. The Vision Fire caused devastating losses but it is also a story of rebirth and regeneration.

As fire sweeps through forest and brushlands, it primes the ecosystem for regeneration. Fire causes old dead foliage as well as newly burned plants to release nutrients and return them to the soil. It promotes new growth by clearing the ground of duff and debris, reducing competition from other plants, and allowing sunlight to reach seedlings. Other than in the bishop-pine forest on Inverness Ridge, where the fire burned the hottest, most of the Vision Fire was of low intensity, and benefited the plants and animals.

Bishop-pine forests are especially well-adapted to fire. In fact, these closed-cone trees depend on fire for survival. Their cones are sealed by a thick resin, which melts and releases the seeds only with intense heat. Once released, bishop-pine seedlings quickly germinate and thrive in the cleared, mineral-rich soil.

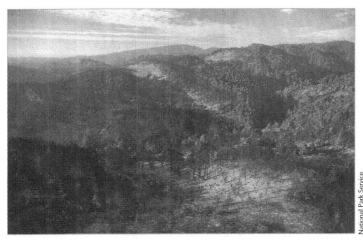

Aftermath of the Vision Fire

Because they burn in large stands and depend on fire as their sole means of regeneration, most bishop pines in one forest are about the same age, all having taken hold after the last burn. Without fire to regenerate the bishop-pine forest, it would eventually die out after about 120 years, having no means of releasing new seedlings. On Inverness Ridge and across the coastal slope, masses of seedlings sprouted beneath the burned trees in the months following the Vision Fire.

The soil's supply of nitrogen—an essential nutrient for plants—vaporizes during a fire. In the carefully orchestrated natural cycle, the first post-fire plants to appear are nitrogen-fixing plants—that is, plants that can turn nitrogen in the air into a water-soluble substance that plants can easily absorb. One such plant is lotus, a ground cover that took hold after the fire in vast carpets. Following lotus, lupine appeared in abundance, and then ceanothus. By the next spring, the burn area was covered in green new growth.

Biologists were primarily concerned about the Vision Fire's effect on animals; however, the burn area buzzed with activity after the fire. Many animals instinctively protect themselves from fire: some leave the area at the first hint of smoke, and others congregate in wet riparian areas that burn less intensely or not at all. Burrowing animals, even those that dig just a few inches beneath the soil, are often sheltered from fire. Salamanders bury themselves underground in the fall, so the Point Reyes population survived the fire well. Red-legged frogs also survived the burn.

Researchers discovered that after the fire, more birds gathered in riparian patches within the burn area than at unburned sites, and species from habitats as diverse as coastal scrub, bishop-pine forest, and marshland all convened in the same protected areas. The year just after the fire, more baby birds hatched in the burn area than anywhere else in the park. The thick new growth, low to the ground, created ideal nesting habitat. Animals that feast on seeds and predatory animals often flock to post-burn areas.

One of the few animals that did suffer from the fire was the Point Reyes mountain beaver. This primitive rodent (*Aplodontia rufa phaea*) is a subspecies of mountain beaver that lives almost exclusively in Point Reyes and burrows in shaded thickets of vegetation. Mature stands of coyote bush provide just the right density, but the vigorous post-burn growth of ceanothus and blackberry was too thick; mountain beavers' primitive kidney doesn't retain enough water for them to survive in more open areas where moisture is less. Biologists estimate that it will take about 20 years for the regenerating coastal scrub to mature into a healthy habitat for mountain beavers.

See the Bayview Trailhead section under Limantour Road Trailheads for trails where you can view the fire's effects and nature's regeneration process.

Opposite page: Indian Beach on Tomales Bay

Human History

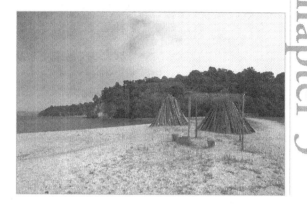

When you walk Point Reyes trails and paddle its waterways, you're following the tracks of many who have come before you—Native Americans wore footpaths through the grasses and navigated fishing crafts in the bays, European galleons landed on the beaches and explorers traveled overland, and dairy ranchers reached their isolated outposts on rough roads and in small schooners. Knowing the rich cultural history of Point Reyes can help you understand and enjoy the landscape it has shaped.

THE FIRST RESIDENTS

Before European explorers and settlers arrived on the Point Reyes peninsula, Coast Miwok lived on this land for thousands of years. More than 100 villages, some with several hundred inhabitants, dotted the point's sloping mesas, the shores of Drakes Estero, and the hills across Tomales Bay. Archeologists believe that more people inhabited the peninsula and the surrounding area in the 16th century than do in the 21st, living off of the wealth of game, fish, and plants this fertile land supported.

Shellmounds near village sites contain bones, tools, shells, and baskets that reveal clues to how Coast Miwok lived. With obsidian arrows, they hunted deer, elk, bear, and mountain lion. Coast Miwok used every part of the animals they killed—bones, antlers, muscle tendons, and furs—and fashioned tools out of natural materials. Bundled tule became building material for the shallow boats they used to fish for salmon, bass, herring, and rock cod in Tomales Bay. From the land, Coast Miwok gathered acorns and supplemented their diet with hazelnuts, young greens, and bulbs. Mussels, clams, and an occasional marine mammal also provided nourishment.

When the first European visitors arrived at Point Reyes, Coast Miwok welcomed them with gifts and ceremonies; the extensive changes these first visits portended would have been impossible to imagine then.

You can learn more about Coast Miwok at Point Reyes by visiting Kule Loklo, a replica of a Coast Miwok village, located at Bear Valley Headquarters (see pages 104–105).

EARLY EUROPEANS

The first Europeans to set foot on the Point Reyes peninsula were most likely Francis Drake (he had not yet been knighted) and his crew in 1579, but Drake's precise landing site is at the center of a controversy that has aroused great passion over the years. Most historians believe Drake careened his ship the *Golden Hinde* at what is today called Drakes Bay for several weeks before returning to his native England. See pages 154–155 for more about the Drake landing site and controversy.

In the late 16th century, the Spanish government in Mexico sent many ships on trading expeditions to Asia, seeking luxuries such as silk, spices, and porcelain. Many such ships passed Point Reyes as they returned by way of the California coast, riding the north winds down to Mexico. In 1595, Sebastián Cermeño, a Portuguese captain commissioned by the Spanish, was en route from the Philippines to Mexico, when fierce winds forced him to seek shelter. He anchored his Manila galleon, loaded with precious cargo, in Drakes Bay and went ashore with most of his crew. A sudden storm swept in and wrecked the *San Agustin*. The boat is thought to still be submerged in the bay.

Cermeño and his crew salvaged a small open launch, and in a great feat of determination and navigational skill, they rowed safely to Mexico. Had the *San Agustin* avoided that disastrous storm, and had Cermeño and his galleon continued down the coast, his place in history may well be quite different. Might he have been the first European to happen upon the San Francisco Bay, almost two centuries before Portolá's overland expedition glimpsed the bay?

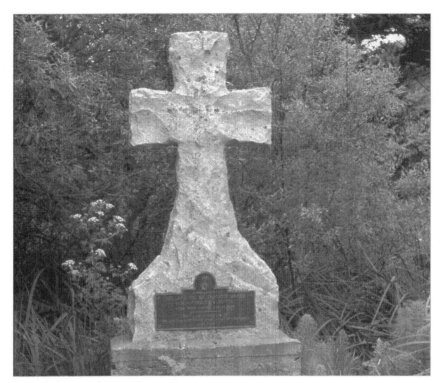

Monument at Drakes Beach

Shards of History

Thousands of shards of Chinese porcelain washed up on the shore of Drakes Bay and in middens on the peninsula expose fascinating evidence of European exploration at Point Reyes. Through comparisons with pieces from kilns in China, some still operating today, researchers have linked patterns, colors, and clay types to specific years. In the late 1570s, when Drake likely landed at Point Reyes, most pottery was made of light clay, decorated with delicate patterns in deep cobalt. Shards of this type found in middens on the peninsula were never immersed in water, and may be from the trunks that the Drake expedition diaries mention having left with Coast Miwok—further evidence that Point Reyes was the site of the much-disputed Drake landing.

Some twenty years after Drake's landing, in the 1590s, China suffered a cobalt shortage and the patterns on exported porcelain were lighter blue in color and less delicate in design, and the clay was of a grayish tint. Archeologists discovered shards of this characteristic pottery on the beaches of Drakes Bay. They probably washed ashore from Cermeño's galleon the *San Agustin*, ship-wrecked in the bay in 1595, known to be carrying hundreds of pieces of Ming dynasty porcelain.

A few years later, one of the survivors of the treacherous return trip to Mexico, Sebastián Vizcaino, made his way back up the California coast a few years later, mapping and naming many landforms along the way. Año Nuevo—known for the elephant seals that spend the winter months there—and Monterey are two of the names that remain today. He reached the waters off the peninsula on January 6, 1603, Día de los Reyes (Day of the Three Kings), and thus recorded the point of land on the map as Punta de los Reyes.

According to journals, the exchanges between European explorers and Coast Miwok living at Point Reyes were peaceful and friendly.

THE MISSIONS

Point Reyes was part of the Spanish colony of Alta California, although the Spaniards never settled the peninsula. In 1817, Franciscan Fathers built Mission San Rafael Arcangel (in what is today the East Marin town of San Rafael) and persuaded thousands of local Native Americans to leave their land and live at the mission. The Fathers baptized them into the Catholic Church and convinced them to take up agriculture. In this unfamiliar setting, removed from their land and way of life, many Coast Miwok contracted and died from European-introduced diseases, particularly smallpox.

MEXICAN RULE AND LAND GRANTS

In 1821, Mexico won independence from Spain, and for the next 27 years, until California became a territory of the United States, Mexico governed Alta California. During that time, the Californios introduced ranching in West Marin; longhorn cattle, used for their hides and tallow rather than their meat, roamed the grasslands. When Mexican civil authorities secularized Mission San Rafael, which had owned most of West Marin, the governors began to dole out large land grants to private citizens for cattle ranching. Coast Miwok received a parcel of land, but it was soon confiscated by settlers, forcing the land's original inhabitants to work on local ranches to earn their livelihood.

The land grants handed out by the government were ill-defined, and land-holders were remarkably casual about their property lines; when owners tried to sell their land, they became tangled in complicated litigation. By the late 1850s, the San Francisco law firm of two brothers, Oscar Shafter and James McMillan Shafter, who had represented several landowners in title cases, had acquired most of the peninsula.

THE DAIRY EMPIRE

Once the Shafter brothers owned most of Point Reyes, they wasted no time in developing a huge dairy enterprise, which would soon become the largest in California. In the mid-1850s, a few families on the peninsula had successfully experimented with making dairy products on a small scale, but the Shafter brothers envisioned a prosperous dairy empire, thriving in the open grasslands and coastal climate of Point Reyes. The long distance to markets in San Francisco seemed an obstacle in those days, but the Shafter brothers foresaw that they could quickly transport cheese and butter to the city by schooner.

When Charles Webb Howard married Oscar Shafter's daughter, he joined the family enterprise, and the three men divided the peninsula among themselves, into 33 ranches. Several ranchers were already grazing dairy cows on Point Reyes, and the Shafters initially signed new leases with them, creating a system of tenant dairy farms. Oscar Shafter and Charles Howard designated their ranches with a letter of the alphabet, from A Ranch at the tip of the headlands to Z Ranch on the summit of Mt. Wittenberg. James Shafter chose names like Drakes Head and Muddy Hollow.

> The location and climate of Point Reyes were key to the success of the dairy industry here. A visitor to the peninsula in the mid-1800s cited "the superior quality of the pasture—the land lying so near the sea, that the dews are heavy and constant, adding great luxuriance to the wild oats and other grains and grasses."

The 1849 Gold Rush brought droves of migrants to California, from the United States and abroad, most of whom were not destined to profit from the precious metal. Many sought other means of making riches from California's natural resources. New arrivals from Ireland, the Azores, and Switzerland became tenant farmers on the Shafters' Point Reyes ranches; many had raised cattle in their homelands. Chinese, Swedish, and Danish immigrants, and many Coast Miwok also worked at the dairies.

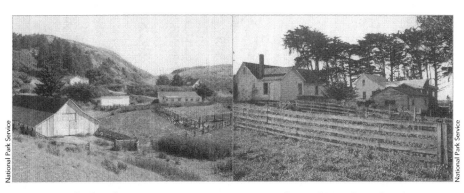

Lake Ranch   Lower Pierce Point Ranch

Without refrigeration, Point Reyes was too far from the city to sell raw milk without spoilage. Butter, however, made the trip well. Point Reyes dairy ranches quickly became celebrated for the quantity and quality of butter they produced. Workers packed 2-pound rolls of butter, shaped by a hand press and stamped "P.R.," into oblong wooden boxes, ready to be shipped by schooner to San Francisco.

Point Reyes butter was lauded by customers in the city, among them the elite Palace Hotel. According to a *San Francisco Chronicle* reporter in 1887: "It is simply perfect, and when you see the name Point Reyes affixed to anything inferior, you may know the trade mark is spurious." In the late 19th century, Point Reyes dairy ranches produced more butter than anywhere else in the state—932,429 pounds in 1867 alone—and dominated the state's dairy industry for decades. The dairies also produced cheese and raised live hogs, all sent to the city by schooner from landing sites on Drakes Estero and Tomales Bay. Marin County ranches launched the California dairy industry, now the largest in the country.

The only piece of the peninsula the Shafter brothers initially sold was the northernmost tip, Tomales Point. Their old friend Solomon Pierce built two ranches on the isolated point and developed a dairy business that surpassed the Shafters'. (See pages 175–176 for more about Pierce Point Ranch, now maintained as an historic site.)

In 1875, the North Pacific Coast Railroad extended its line up the east shore of Tomales Bay, en route to North Coast timber operations. James Shafter, president of the railroad company, invested heavily in this transportation novelty, and, for a time, the peninsula's butter, cheese, and hogs reached the city by rail. Shafter's investment eventually sent him into debt; the Northwestern Pacific Railroad (as it was then called) abandoned the line through Point Reyes in 1933.

NEW OWNERS

The Point Reyes dairy industry began to decline in the first decades of the 20th century, faced with competition from new and improved dairies in other parts of the state. In addition, the land itself presented obstacles to ranching. Early Anglo settlers arriving at Point Reyes did not realize that the perennially green, treeless moors of Point Reyes had been cultivated for over hundreds of years: Coast Miwok had burned, pruned, and harvested the land, and herds of tule elk had grazed the hillsides. Without this management, coyote bush, poison oak, and scrub thickets encroached on ranches, especially on Inverness Ridge.

As the Shafter/Howard clan fell deeper into debt, their monopoly on Point Reyes land began to deteriorate. They were forced to sell their ranches, the majority to the tenant farmers who ran them. The Shafter's alphabet ranches took on the names of the Irish, Portuguese, and Italian-Swiss families who acquired them; some of the families—McClure, Kehoe, Mendoza, Grossi—remain today. The first of the Shafter/Howard land was sold in 1919, and by 1939, the family held no title on the peninsula.

Point Reyes ranchers encountered difficult times in the ensuing years. Bootlegging and rum-running were common practice on the isolated peninsula during Prohibition, and some ranches depended on liquor smuggling as their only source of income. During the lean years of the Depression, many ranchers diversified their production with beef cattle, chicken, and eggs.

CREATION OF THE NATIONAL SEASHORE

The National Park Service had its eye on Point Reyes as early as 1935, when it recommended purchase of 53,000 acres for recreational use. At $45 per acre, the price sounds like a bargain today, but it was a huge sum in Depression years. The survey and the recommendation were shelved for two decades.

Meanwhile, conservationists succeeded in preserving a few parcels of land as county parks: part of Drakes Beach in 1938, McClures Beach in 1942, and Shell Beach in 1945. The county later turned them over to the National Park Service and California State Parks.

But alongside these conservation successes, people looking to profit from the land and natural resources of Point Reyes were quickly compromising the peninsula's rich natural beauty and diversity. As dairy ranching on Inverness Ridge came to an end, ranchers looked for other business ventures. In 1947, the hopeful owner of Lake Ranch granted an oil lease to drill on his land, but National Exploration Company found no black gold. Several land owners sold timber rights when Marin County placed a tax on standing timber, and in 1958, Sweet Lumber Company began felling Douglas-firs on Inverness Ridge. Developers were dreaming up grandiose plans for other parts of the peninsula, including a subdivision on Limantour Spit with half-acre homesites, a golf course, and a boat harbor. A 1959 highway plan calling for a multi-lane thoroughfare from San Rafael to Point Reyes Station threatened to bring to an end the peninsula's isolation and pave the way for urbanization.

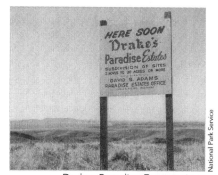

Drakes Paradise Estates sign

The creation of Point Reyes National Seashore was the result of citizen activism and the foresight and perseverance of a few visionary leaders in the federal government and local conservation organizations. In 1956, the National

Park Service conducted a recreation survey of the entire Pacific Coast, and their interest once again came to rest on Point Reyes. With the threats to its existence as an undeveloped area seemingly imminent, Marin conservationists and key officials in the National Park Service recognized the need for immediate action to preserve Point Reyes. Conservation-minded community members rallied together under the theme of "Point Reyes...An Island in Time." A partnership between the Sierra Club and the Point Reyes National Seashore Foundation produced a book by the same name, written by local environmental writer Harold Gilliam. Supporters flooded the newspapers with articles urging people to back the national seashore.

In Washington, Representative Clem Miller and Senator Clair Engle introduced Seashore legislation bills in Congress in 1959, calling for acquisition of 53,000 acres. In April 1960, members of a Senate committee flew over the peninsula and were stunned with the beauty of the land. Arguments from Park Service Director Conrad Wirth for the "intrinsic natural beauties" of Point Reyes, and Secretary of the Interior Stewart Udall's encouragement convinced Congress that Point Reyes was worthy of national seashore status.

But not everyone wanted to see the peninsula become federal property. In Washington and locally, park supporters and opponents came head-to-head in a complex controversy over the creation of the national seashore. Developers forged ahead with their plans for the Drakes Beach Estates subdivision, leveling hills, grading roads, and beginning construction on homes. They ran ads in the local papers that encouraged people to "Option your Drakes Bay lot now! You can put a 'hold' on a fabulous Drakes Bay homesite until you're SURE it will remain private property!"

Many ranchers contested the creation of the national seashore, being opposed to turning over to the federal government the land their families had lived on and worked for generations. The Marin Conservation League, a prominent pro-park organization, argued for the coexistence of ranching and recreation, emphasizing that "as true conservationists we want to preserve dairying in this area and will do what we can to promote the health of this industry." The league suggested the solution that ultimately brought about compromise, in which existing ranchers were allowed to continue ranching with long-term leases on 26,000 acres of land. The compromise also allowed RCA and AT&T to maintain their radio facilities on the point. After extensive negotiations, on September 13, 1962, President John F. Kennedy signed the bill authorizing 53,000 acres of Point Reyes National Seashore.

The authorization was an important step, but the national seashore was still not secure: Congress appropriated only enough money to buy a small portion of the land, so after a few purchases, the funds were used up. Land prices continued to rise and developers were still voraciously eyeing park-designated lots. In

1972, another citizen action campaign, "Save Our Seashore," led by Marin County Supervisor Peter Behr, succeeded in getting President Nixon to authorize funds to purchase the remaining acreage.

The 10-year delay proved auspicious, as park planning and public sentiment changed significantly during those years. In the early 1960s, National Park Service guidelines allowed for more organized and motorized recreation development in national seashores than in national parks. At Point Reyes National Seashore, plans called for a network of roads and facilities to accommodate motor boats, dune buggies, campers, trailers, and thousands of cars. Boating, golf, softball, deep-sea sport fishing, and other activities were all part of the original idea for the park.

However, by the time the last parcel of Point Reyes became part of the national seashore, the Park Service had begun to rethink how parks should be used. A growing environmental consciousness led people to value preservation as much as or more than recreation, and locals wanted to preserve the natural state of the peninsula and its unique heritage as much as possible. The only major construction implemented from the original park plans was Limantour Road.

The tide that brought changes in the earlier plans for the park continued rising, and the concept of the seashore turned more and more toward one where preservation triumphed over recreational development. In 1976, the National Park Service proposed designating 5000 acres of Point Reyes as wilderness. In a familiar tradition, citizens once again banded together in support of a more ambitious proposal, which resulted in the creation of 32,000 acres of wilderness within the park. In 1985, the wilderness area was named for Congressman Phillip Burton of San Francisco, who was responsible for more than doubling the wilderness acreage in the national park system and for the creation of the Golden Gate National Recreation Area.

Loss and Legacy

Had the debates about Point Reyes National Seashore dragged on any longer, the Point Reyes peninsula might have looked very different today. Within a couple of years of the seashore bill's authorization, tragic events befell three instrumental figures: Congressman Clem Miller, a key supporter of the seashore, died in a plane crash on October 7, 1962, just weeks after President Kennedy signed the legislation. Less than a year later, Kennedy planned to visit Point Reyes, but a last-minute change to his itinerary sent him to Dallas, where he was shot to death; he never saw for himself the land he had helped save. Senator Clair Engle, who had pushed the seashore legislation through the Senate, died of cancer on July 30, 1964. Less than two years after the long battle for the seashore was won, all three of its champions had died.

LAND AROUND THE PARK

Development plans for park-slated land were minor in comparison to the vision for greater West Marin. In the 1960s and 1970s, during the Point Reyes National Seashore acquisition process, the West Marin General Plan, as proposed by the pro-growth Board of Supervisors, seriously threatened the agricultural lands surrounding the park and the rural way of life they supported.

The general plan called for an extensive highway system connecting urban East Marin to the rural coast, including a multi-lane thoroughfare from San Rafael to Point Reyes Station. Pastures and open space would be converted to shopping centers, car dealerships, golf courses, and urban settlements of

MARIN AGRICULTURAL LAND TRUST

Imagine a city of 150,000 people on the shores of Tomales Bay, homes marching up hillsides, bayside resorts in place of oyster farms, and roads crisscrossing cattle pastures, connecting golf courses and mini-malls. In the 1960s and 1970s, some Marin County planners did envision this, and concerned local citizens set to work to be sure that their dreams never materialized.

In the late 1970s, two local conservationists—activist Phyllis Faber and rancher Ellen Straus—began to look for a way to avoid the development of West Marin ranches and the loss of the agricultural lifestyle. They came up with the idea of an unprecedented local land trust. After many meetings between wary ranchers and conservationists, in 1980 an unusual coalition of farm and environmental leaders formed the Marin Agricultural Land Trust (MALT), dedicated to permanently preserving Marin County farmland while allowing continued agricultural use of the land.

More than two decades since its creation, MALT has protected more than 30,000 acres of agricultural land and nearly 50 farms and ranches. What began as a visionary experiment has proved a long-term success. MALT has set West Marin on a dramatically different path from the one the county had envisioned in the 1960s, significantly influencing the environment, economics, lifestyle, and landscape of the area around Point Reyes National Seashore.

How has MALT achieved such success? The land trust buys conservation easements from ranchers that prohibit subdivision and nonagricultural development of their lands. The money ranchers receive helps them to pay property and estate taxes and to fund modernization projects. This method of preserving land has become a model for the nation, and MALT is one of the oldest and largest agricultural preservation organizations in the United States.

MALT offers visitors to Point Reyes many ways to connect with the rural past and present of West Marin. You can find out about local ranching history with

150,000 people. A junior college at Millerton Point on Tomales Bay, an estate development on Black Mountain, cluster housing in Olema, and apartments in the marshes of Tomales Bay would house and serve the population. More than 130,000 acres of productive dairy lands were at risk, and the plan included no viable proposals for water or sewage. Land speculators made eager by the prospect of development bought up land on the east shore of Tomales Bay, inflating land prices and thus jeopardizing the full acquisition of the national seashore.

Again, citizen action triumphed: concerned local residents changed the face of the Board of Supervisors by electing anti-development members. The supervisors adopted a new plan that limited urbanization to the eastern part of the county.

an audio-cassette-tape driving tour, available at national seashore visitor centers and from the MALT website. An annual Harvest Day at the Farm celebrates the bounty of local farms with a full day of festivities—barbequed chicken, oysters, music, pony rides, pumpkins, buttermaking, weaving, and more. Every spring, *plein air* painters exhibit their works at *Ranches & Rolling Hills,* a landscape art show and sale that benefits MALT. MALT tours of local ranches and farms offer an up-close view of everything from local milk and grass-fed beef production to organic vegetables, olive groves, and vineyards. You'll learn more about West Marin food production and enjoy the end product—cheese, oysters, beef, olive oil, and more. Find out more about MALT, the activities they offer, and membership at www.malt.org or by calling (415) 663-1158.

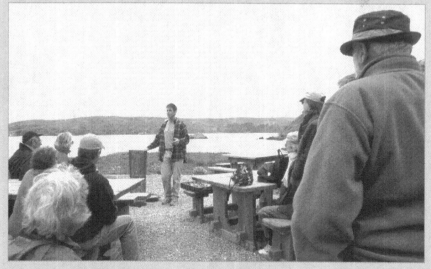

MALT tour of Hog Island Oyster Company

To help maintain agricultural land use, in 1972 they voted to restrict zoning to 60-acre-minumum parcels in West Marin.

In the late 1970s, local community leaders began to look for a more permanent solution to the problem of development of West Marin agricultural lands. An unusual coalition of ranchers and environmentalists came together to form the Marin Agricultural Land Trust (MALT), which has proved to be a long-term success in preserving ranching in West Marin.

Opposite page: Birding on the Tomales Point Trail

Visiting Point Reyes and the Surrounding Area

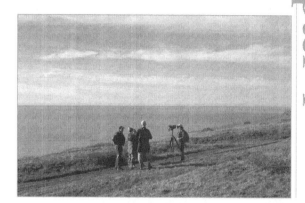

Chapter 4

VISITOR INFORMATION

DIRECTIONS TO POINT REYES AND SURROUNDING AREA

These directions take you to the towns of Olema and Point Reyes Station and to Point Reyes National Seashore headquarters at Bear Valley. To reach other trailheads and locations in this book, see individual sections.

From Highway 101 there are two routes to the park. From San Francisco, the shortest route is via Sir Francis Drake Boulevard. Take the Sir Francis Drake exit from 101 in San Anselmo and head west on Sir Francis Drake Boulevard through several towns, including Greenbrae, San Anselmo, and Fairfax (where you may encounter a fair amount of traffic), and Samuel P. Taylor State Park to reach Highway 1 at Olema (about 21 miles from Highway 101). To reach Point Reyes Station, turn right at the stop sign and follow Highway 1 north for 2 miles. To reach Bear Valley headquarters in Point Reyes National Seashore, turn right on Highway 1 and then left immediately on Bear Valley Rd. Continue 0.5 mile to the visitor center road and turn left and go 0.2 mile to a large paved parking area.

Lucas Valley Road is a more scenic route from Highway 101 (and more convenient for travelers coming from the north). Exit on Lucas Valley Road and follow the winding road west for several miles to Nicasio Valley Road. Turn right, pass the town of Nicasio and the Nicasio Reservoir, and turn left on the Point Reyes-Petaluma Road. Continue around the reservoir, beneath the eastern slopes of Black Mountain, and turn right at the next stop sign to reach Highway 1 at Point Reyes Station in 3 miles. Turn left on Highway 1 and follow it through town.

To reach Olema, continue south on Highway 1 for 2 miles. To reach Bear Valley headquarters in Point Reyes National Seashore, turn right on Sir Francis Drake Blvd. just after crossing the green bridge at the southern edge of town and go 0.7 mile to Bear Valley Rd.. Turn left and continue 1.7 miles to the visitor center road; turn right and go 0.2 mile to a large paved parking area.

The most scenic route to Point Reyes is Highway 1. Take the Stinson Beach/Highway 1 exit from Highway 101, and follow Highway 1 along the coast and up the Olema Valley (about 26 miles from the Golden Gate Bridge to Olema). Although quite a bit longer because of the narrow, winding road, this coastal route takes in spectacular scenery.

Approaching from Petaluma and points north, take the Tomales–Petaluma Road to the town of Tomales. Turn left on Highway 1 and follow it along Tomales Bay to Point Reyes Station.

West Marin roads are narrow and winding. Numerous bicyclists and motorcyclists travel these roads, especially on weekends. Please drive with extreme caution, pass only in legally designated sections and when you are certain all is clear, and use turnouts when necessary.

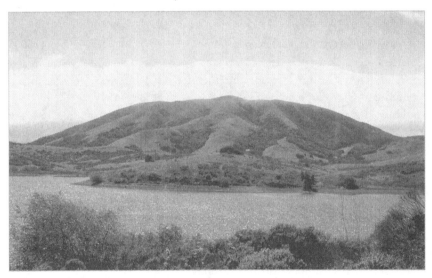

Black Mountain across Nicasio Reservoir

During heavy storms, some West Marin roads may be closed due to flooding or fallen trees. Call Caltrans at (800) 427-7623 or (415) 557-3755.

Getting there by bus:

Golden Gate Transit
(415) 923-2000
Bus #63 goes from Marin City to Audubon Canyon Ranch Bolinas Lagoon Preserve on weekends while the preserve is open.

West Marin Stagecoach
(415) 526-3239, www.marin-stagecoach.org
Weekday service from San Anselmo to Samuel P. Taylor State Park, Olema, Point Reyes Station, and Inverness; from Marin City to Muir Beach, Stinson Beach, and Bolinas.

HAZARDS AND SAFETY ADVICE

POISON OAK

The oily residue that coats poison oak leaves and branches can result in a blistering, itchy rash on some people. After contact with the oil, a rash may develop in mere hours or in a week or two. The oily residue is hard to wash off and can be transferred to skin from clothing, fur, and other materials (dogs are notorious carriers). You can contract the oil at any time of year: shiny green leaves in summer, brilliant red fall foliage, and spare sticks in winter are all potent.

Poison oak grows in most every habitat at Point Reyes—forests, riparian areas, open chaparral, and coastal bluffs—but if you exercise caution, you can avoid touching it: keep your hands, feet, and backpack close to your body when walking narrow trails, and watch for overhanging branches on wide trails. Most importantly, know what to look for! Poison oak's appearance can vary deceptively: its shiny, lobed leaves may be very large or very small, and they most often grow in clusters of three but some variations grow in fives.

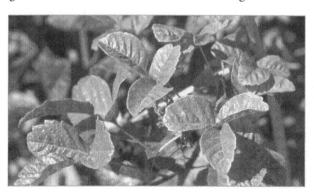

Poison oak

If you come into contact with poison oak, the best antidote is to wash the contaminated area thoroughly with soap. People who are especially sensitive may want to try a soap that is specifically formulated to combat the plant's oil, such as Tecnu Oak-n-Ivy Cleanser or Ivy Block. Be sure to wash your clothes, too.

STINGING NETTLE

Stinging nettle's leaves and stem are covered with tiny hairs filled with formic acid. When you brush against the plant, the acid releases onto your skin, causing a painful stinging or tingling sensation that can last as long as a day. In spring, nettle plants along moist, shady trails become tall and rangy.

Horses are especially sensitive to stinging nettle. In extreme cases, excessive contact with the plant can cause anaphylactic shock in horses and possibly death. Heed trail closures, as trails that are no longer maintained by the park may be overgrown with nettle. For the most up-to-date information about trail closures, check with the Bear Valley Visitor Center.

If you're not sure what stinging nettle looks like, identify it at the Bear Valley Visitor Center before your trip.

TICKS

Second to poison oak, ticks are probably the most common aggravation you'll encounter at Point Reyes, especially in spring and summer. When you brush against trailside grasses and shrubs, these tiny teardrop-shaped pests (about an eighth of an inch long) hitch onto your clothing and make their way to an open patch of skin.

If you are bitten by a tick, use tweezers to pull it out, taking care to remove any mouth parts. Do not touch the tick, since the "juice" also can transmit the disease. Wash the bite area and your hands with warm water and soap and apply an antiseptic. Contact your physician if the mouth or head breaks off and remains under your skin, or if you experience fatigue, muscle and joint pain, chills, fever, or headaches.

Some ticks transmit Lyme disease, although only 1 to 2 percent of ticks in California are infected with the disease. Try to avoid narrow, overgrown trails during tick season. Wearing long pants (preferably light-colored, so that ticks will be visible), and tucking them into your socks can help avoid tick bites. Some insect repellents are effective against ticks. After hiking, check your body for ticks, particularly in warm, moist places.

GIARDIA

Water in streams and lakes in the Point Reyes area may contain *Giardia lamblia*, a protozoan that causes severe intestinal illness and discomfort. Don't drink directly from any untreated water sources and always carry plenty of treated water with you. Water at Glen, Coast, and Sky camps is potable, but not at Wildcat Camp.

MOUNTAIN LIONS

Mountain lions live at Point Reyes, but it is unlikely that you will encounter one of these elusive animals, and an attack is even less likely.

If you meet a mountain lion on the trail, here are a few basic rules to follow:
- Do not run—running away stimulates the cat's predatory instincts.
- Do not turn your back—make eye contact and back away slowly from the animal.
- Do not bend down—you'll look like a four-legged prey.
- Pick up pets or small children immediately (without bending down).
- Stand upright and make yourself look larger by raising your arms above your head or opening your jacket, if you are wearing one.
- Throw stones, branches, or whatever you can reach without crouching or turning your back.
- If approached, wave your arms and speak firmly or shout.
- If attacked, fight back aggressively; since a mountain lion usually tries to bite the head or neck, try to remain standing and face the attacking animal.

SAFETY ON THE TRAIL
- Do not shortcut switchbacks; shortcuts cause erosion and damage trails.
- Stay on trails to avoid poison oak, stinging nettle, and ticks.
- Be prepared for wind, rain, fog, and sunshine. Wear layered clothing.
- Carry your own water; potable water is available only at visitor centers and some campgrounds.
- Do not drink from streams; the protozoan *Giardia lamblia* can cause severe intestinal illness.
- Stay away from cliff edges and do not climb cliff walls. Cliffs are unstable and highly erosive.
- When you meet a horse on the trail, step to the downhill side, greet the rider, and do not touch the animal.

SAFETY AT THE BEACH
- Be aware of the tide. High tide and unscalable cliffs can trap you on a pocket beach. Check the tide tables posted at visitor centers before you go.
- No lifeguards are stationed at beaches.
- Strong currents, treacherous surf, and cold water make swimming and wading in the ocean beaches (Point Reyes North and South, Abbotts, Kehoe, and McClures) extremely dangerous.
- Keep an eye on the surf even when you are on the beach: sleeper waves can surprise you and knock you down without notice (and can even carry away an unleashed dog).
- Loose soil and rocks make beach cliffs unstable and unsafe. Do not climb cliff walls, and stay away from cliff edges.

We think of logging, roads, and dams all as destructive to nature, but as recreationists, we also affect the natural environment. By treating animals, plants, and other humans in natural areas with respect and care we can lessen our impact and preserve precious habitats.

- Do not feed or chase wildlife.
- Stay at least 300 feet from marine mammals. If you notice that your presence disturbs animals, move away immediately.
- If you encounter a solitary harbor seal or elephant seal, do not touch it.
- Do not tromp on or pick flowers or plants.
- Stay on trails to prevent erosion as well as to avoid poison oak, stinging nettle, and ticks. Avoid areas that are closed for erosion control or revegetation.
- Don't cut switchbacks or make shortcuts. Don't create new trails to avoid muddy sections.
- Pack out your trash. Leave no trace!
- Keep your noise to a minimum.
- Respect dog regulations. Dogs' markings disturb wildlife and interfere with wildlife habitat.
- Don't allow your dog to chase wildlife.

OUTDOOR ACTIVITIES

This section introduces you to the various activities the Point Reyes area offers. Some activities receive only a brief overview here, such as hiking, biking, and horseback riding, because the trails they follow are described in detail in the regional sections of the book. Kayaking, on the other hand, is given full treatment here, from outfitters to launch sites and overnight camping.

For driving directions to the trails and beaches mentioned below, see the appropriate trailheads in Chapters 5 and 6. Also see the locator map at the front of the book.

HIKING

Point Reyes National Seashore and adjacent parks and recreation areas provide miles of trails through an extraordinary range of environments. In the seashore alone, there are more than 140 miles of trails. Most are well signed and generally easy to follow, although you should be aware that the mileage posted on trail signs is not always correct.

Tomales Bay and Samuel P. Taylor state parks, Golden Gate National Recreation Area, and the Audubon Canyon Ranch Bolinas Lagoon Preserve also offer possibilities for full-day hikes and short walks.

See the following chapters for trips and more specific trail information.

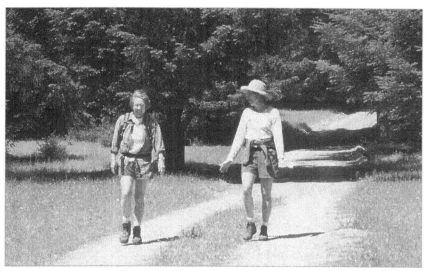
Hikers on Stewart Trail at Firtop

BIKING

Bikes are allowed on over 35 miles of trail within Point Reyes National Seashore. See the maps in this book to find out which trails allow bikes. The Bear Valley Visitor Center also provides a map that shows permissible bike routes. The Bolinas Ridge Trail, in Golden Gate National Recreation Area, is a great route for bikes, and a few trails in Samuel P. Taylor State Park are open to bikes.

Below you'll find pertinent information and a brief outline of bike routes; turn to the corresponding chapters about individual parks for detailed descriptions of these routes.

Point Reyes National Seashore
Bear Valley Trail
Distance: 3.1 miles one-way

Open to bikes for the first 3.1 miles, the Bear Valley Trail is smooth and mostly level, other than a gentle ascent at Divide Meadow. At the junction with the Glen Trail, you can lock your bike at racks provided if you want to continue on foot to the coast, to Glen Camp, or to other destinations. Families and those who want a leisurely ride will enjoy this popular route. See Trip 1.

Coast Trail
Distance: 2.8 miles one-way to Coast Camp

From the trailhead near the Point Reyes hostel to Coast Camp, the Coast Trail is a level, easy ride on a smooth trail, sandy in spots. See Trip 14.

Marshall Beach
Distance: 1.2 miles one-way; additional 5-mile round trip possible
The route to Marshall Beach begins from the parking area on a wide, level trail. You soon descend rather steeply to Tomales Bay on a gravelly trail. Bicyclists who want a longer ride can begin at the intersection of Pierce Point and Duck Cove/Marshall Beach roads for an extra 2.5 scenic miles each way on a dirt road. See Trip 21.

Estero Trail
Distance: 4 miles one-way to Sunset Beach; 4.7 miles one-way to Drakes Head
The Estero Trail to Drakes Head or Sunset Beach makes a great trip for more experienced riders. The trail is rutted and rough in spots and often muddy in the wet season. See Trip 18.

Stewart Trail
Distance: 6.4 miles one-way
A wide, well-graded dirt road from the Five Brooks Trailhead to the coast at Wildcat Camp. See Trip 27.

Inverness Ridge Trail
Distance: 2.8 one-way
This trail begins as a wide dirt road at the Bayview Trailhead. After about a mile, the trail becomes a singletrack and climbs and descends along the ridge to reach Point Reyes Hill and Mt. Vision. A great ride, recommended for more experienced riders who are comfortable with sharp turns and narrow trails. See Trip 12.

Golden Gate National Recreation Area
Bolinas Ridge Trail
Distance: 11 miles one-way
Extremely popular with mountain bikers, this wide trail follows the crest of Bolinas Ridge, gradually but steadily gaining in elevation from the trailhead on Sir Francis Drake to the other end at Alpine Road. You must dismount to pass through cattle gates, and ruts gouge trail in many spots, but the views and pastoral scenery are worth it. See Trip 35.

Samuel P. Taylor State Park
Cross Marin Trail
Distance: 3.4 miles one-way from main park campground to Platform Bridge.
This shaded, paved, and level path along Lagunitas/Papermill Creek is great for families. See Trip 38.

Barnabe and Ridge trails
Distance: 5.7-mile loop

Steep climbs and descents on singletracks and dirt roads make this trip to Barnabe Mountain lots of fun. See Trip 41.

Bike Regulations
- No off-trail riding.
- Do not carry or walk bikes on hiking-only trails.
- Speed limit is 15 miles per hour; slow down on blind curves.
- Bikes yield to horses and hikers.
- Alert other trail users of your approach and indicate how many riders follow.
- Helmets are strongly recommended.

KAYAKING

Tomales Bay and Drakes Estero provide superb spots for kayaking adventures in and around Point Reyes National Seashore and offer unique views of the scenery and wildlife.

Outfitters
Blue Waters Kayaking is the only kayak outfitter that operates on Tomales Bay (they recently merged with Tamal Sea Kayaking). Blue Waters is located in Marshall, on the east side of the bay, about 8 miles north of Point Reyes Station. They offer rentals, instructional classes, full-moon paddles, guided tours, and overnight trips on Tomales Bay and nearby waterways for all levels of paddlers. Open every day, 9 A.M. to 6 P.M. (415) 663-1743. www.bwkayak.com.

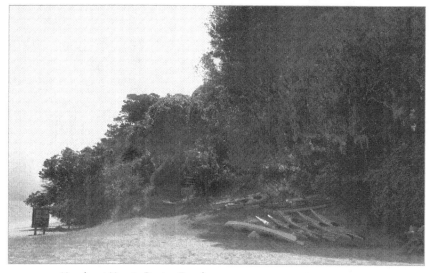

Kayaks at Hearts Desire Beach

(**Blue Waters** allows rentals of open-decked kayaks to people with no previous experience, but closed-deck boats require a class or certification.)

Exploring Tomales Bay
With a rental boat or with your own kayak, you can explore Tomales Bay. As the fog burns off and the sun slowly warms the air, watch osprey soar overhead and dive for fish, look for double-crested cormorant nests on Hog Island, and steer your kayak close to shore to study the rich collage of vegetation that thrives on the steep bayside cliffs. Mornings are best for kayaking on the bay, before the afternoon breeze picks up.

You can launch your own kayak from several sites on Tomales Bay's east and west shores.

Tomales Bay, East Side
For east-side access, take Highway 1 north from Point Reyes Station.

Millerton Point, Tomales Bay State Park
Driving Directions: Follow Highway 1 north from Point Reyes Station for 4.5 miles. Turn left into the parking area, marked by several large eucalyptus trees.
Regulations: No fee, no overnight camping or parking
Launch site: You have to carry your kayak about 100 yards from the parking lot to a small beach. Low tide reveals mudflats beyond the sand, so plan your launch and pullout for high tide. No overnight parking is allowed in Tomales Bay State Park.

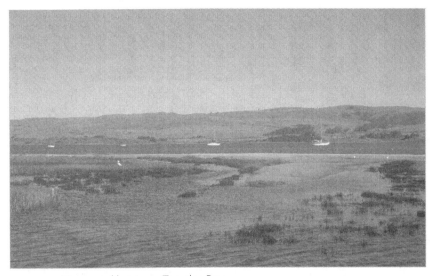

Heron and boats on Tomales Bay

Blue Waters Kayaking

Driving Directions: Follow Highway 1 north from Point Reyes Station for 8 miles. Just beyond the Marshall Boat Yard, you'll see kayaks and a small building on the west side of the road.

Regulations: No fee for private launch

Launch site: This rental outfitter allows private launching from their beach, as long as you don't get in the way of their customers.

Miller County Park

Driving Directions: Follow Highway 1 north from Point Reyes Station for about 12 miles. Look for a small sign on the west side of the highway.

Regulations: Day and overnight use fees

Launch site: You'll find a cement-grade boat launch and day and overnight parking here. Restrooms available. (415) 499-6387.

Lawson's Landing

Driving Directions: Follow Highway 1 north from Point Reyes Station to the town of Tomales. Turn left on Dillon Beach Road; after 4 miles, the road reaches the beach and turns left. Continue to Lawson's Landing at the end of the road.

Regulations: Fee for boat launch and camping

Launch site: Lawson's Landing provides boat launching and camping facilities, and the beach is a popular spot for clammers. Restrooms and water available. Lawson's Landing is close to the mouth of Tomales Bay, where strong currents and winds, and choppy water can make paddling difficult. (707) 878-2443.

Tomales Bay, West Side

West-side access to Tomales Bay is from Sir Francis Drake Highway.

Hearts Desire Beach, Tomales Bay State Park

Driving Directions: Go south on Highway 1 from Point Reyes Station and turn right on Sir Francis Drake Blvd. Continue 2.5 miles beyond Inverness to Pierce Point Road. Veer right and follow it a little over a mile to the signed entrance on the right.

Regulations: Day-use fee. No overnight parking.

Launch site: You must carry your boat a short distance from the parking lot to the launching area on the sand, taking care to avoid the clearly designated swimming area.

Drakes Estero

Blue Waters Kayaking leads trips to Drakes Estero, but if you have your own boat, you can explore this wildlife haven at your leisure. Along with unique water-level views of the surrounding landscape, you have a good chance of seeing harbor seals, white pelicans, bat rays, and leopard sharks.

Driving Directions: Go south on Highway 1 from Point Reyes Station and turn right on Sir Francis Drake Highway. Continue through Inverness to the Pierce Point Road junction. Bear left to stay on Sir Francis Drake. Turn left about 3 miles past the junction, on a road signed to JOHNSON'S OYSTER COMPANY.

Regulations: Off-limits to paddlers during harbor-seal pupping season, between March 15 and June 30. No fishing. No motorized boats. No camping or overnight parking.

Launch Site: A small beach at Johnson's Oyster Company provides a launch site and a good view of the oyster harvest. Always check the tide tables before setting out: at low tide boats can ground on mudflats.

BOAT-IN CAMPING

The national seashore allows boat-in camping at several beaches along the west side of Tomales Bay, beginning north of Indian Beach. You must have an advance reservation permit. You can reserve up to three months in advance (to the day) by calling (415) 663-8054 between 9 A.M. and 2 P.M., Monday through Friday; by coming to Bear Valley Visitor Center in person, seven days a week; or by faxing your reservation to (415) 464-5149 using the park fax form.

TOMALES BAY FROM YOUR KAYAK

The narrow finger of Tomales Bay—12 miles long and only about a mile wide—extends between the Point Reyes peninsula and the mainland, and supports numerous species of wildlife. Coho salmon, steelhead trout, herring, osprey, cormorants, herons, and egrets all depend on the bay's waters, which are protected by the Gulf of the Farallones National Marine Sanctuary. As you paddle the bay and scan its shoreline hills, remember that the wildlife share their habitat not only with recreation, but also with commercial fishing and oyster farming on the bay, and agricultural production on the surrounding lands. These pursuits all affect water quality in the bay, in the 200-plus–acre watershed, and in the six creeks that empty into this brackish estuary.

Paddling on Tomales Bay is the ideal way to see some of the birds that live and feed there. About 25,000 waterbirds visit Tomales Bay each winter, drawn to the abundance of food in its waters. **Surf scoters** swarm over eelgrass beds, stripping herring eggs from the blades or tearing off blades to feast on the roe. You might also see **black brants** grazing in eelgrass beds during March and April. These marine geese, about the size of mallard ducks, fly overhead in long, graceful lines as they migrate north from Baja. **Double-crested cormorants** nest on

Phone reservations require payment by credit card, due at the time you make the reservation. Permits cost $12 per night per site for up to six people, $25 for seven to 14 people, and $35 for 15 to 25 people. No refunds are given for any reason.

Pick up your permit at the visitor center before beginning your trip. If you arrive after the visitor center has closed, you will find your permit in the after-hours box on the information board in front of the building.

Most beaches are small stretches of sand backed by steep cliffs or sloping coastal hillsides. They are subject to tidal influences, so be sure to bring your boat onto the beach, far from the water's edge, and choose your beach carefully if you don't want to wade through mud the next morning to reach the water.

You must provide your own "human waste facilities" at all Tomales Bay beaches except Marshall and Tomales beaches, which provide pit toilets. This means that if you don't bring a porta-potty, you can't camp on the beach. No potable water is available at any of the beaches. Check with the seashore for updates, because some beaches are subject to seasonal closures.

No overnight parking for boat-in campers is allowed in Point Reyes National Seashore or in Tomales Bay State Park. You must launch from a site outside the parks to begin your trip. See the above list of launch sites on Tomales Bay east and west shores.

Hog Island, making the island an unpleasant stop for the kayakers who used to picnic there. Also look for **loons**, including common, pacific, and red-throated, who flock to the bay.

Shorebirds gather in the mudflats at the north and south ends of the bay. **Marbled godwits** prefer sandy areas at the north end and on into Bodega Harbor. Look for clusters of **willets, sandpipers, killdeer, dunlins,** and **black-bellied plovers** along the shoreline, but take care not to disturb these sensitive birds.

You'll likely see **great** and **snowy egrets**, and **great blue herons** from nearby colonies at Bolinas Lagoon, Bear Valley, and Drakes Estero foraging in mudflats. **Osprey** frequently descend from their nests on Inverness Ridge to fish in the bay. Keep a close eye on these phenomenal birds as they soar overhead. With their binocular-like eyes, osprey spot their prey from high above the water. As they dive to make their catch, they triangulate to predict the position of the fish when they reach it, adjusting for movement and refraction. Despite the complications of their hunting method, osprey are some of the most successful predators among birds, nabbing their victim about 60 percent of the time.

Boat-in Camp Regulations

- No overnight camping on Hog Island (east side), Pelican Point, Hearts Desire Beach, or Indian Beach; South Blue Gum Beach closed to overnight camping from March 15 to June 30.
- Groups of more than 15 people must camp on Marshall or Tomales beaches.
- Fires require a permit and are allowed only on beaches, away from vegetation (pick up a free permit at the Bear Valley Visitor Center).
- All waste (including human) must be removed.
- No dogs or other pets allowed.
- Store food in storage lockers to protect it from animals.
- Do not feed wildlife.
- Pack out all trash.
- Respect your camp neighbors: observe quiet hours, from sunset to sunrise.
- Camping outside designated campsites or without a permit is illegal.
- Four-night per visit limit; maximum of 30 nights per year.
- No firearms or fireworks.

HORSEBACK RIDING

Point Reyes National Seashore is a horse-friendly recreation area: horses are allowed on all trails in the seashore, except on weekends and holidays, when the Meadow and Old Pine trails and the Bear Valley Trail from the trailhead to the Glen Trail are closed to horses.

Horses are allowed on all Golden Gate National Recreation Area trails covered in this book and on most trails in Samuel P. Taylor State Park. Trails in Tomales Bay State Park and the Audubon Canyon Ranch Bolinas Lagoon Preserve are not open to horses.

Five Brooks Ranch, located at the Five Brooks Trailhead on Highway 1, 3.5 miles south of Olema, offers guided rides, horse rentals, horse boarding, and hayrides. Open every day, 9 A.M. to 5 P.M. Reservations recommended. (415) 663-1570. www.fivebrooks.com.

At **Chanslor Ranch** in Bodega Bay you can bring your own horse or take a lesson or a guided ride with theirs. They also offer horse boarding and care. (707) 875-3333.

Stewart Horse Camp on Highway 1, 3 miles south of Olema, provides campsites for equestrians. (415) 663-1362.

In Samuel P. Taylor State Park, **Devils Gulch Horse Camp** has one equestrian group campsite for up to 20 people and 16 horses.

BEACHCOMBING AND SWIMMING

As you might expect at a national seashore, Point Reyes beaches are superb. Some you can drive to and others you must reach by trail—foot, bike, or horse. **Limantour, Drakes, Kehoe, McClures, Marshall,** and **Palomarin** beaches,

OPEN WATER ESSENTIALS

Safety on the water

- Check the tide tables before you go by calling Bear Valley Visitor Center (415) 464-5100 or Tomales Bay State Park (415) 669-1140; low tide exposes mudflats on Tomales Bay and Drakes Estero and you might become stuck; near the mouth of Tomales Bay and Drakes Estero, incoming and outgoing tides create strong and hazardous currents.
- Always wear a personal flotation device (life jacket) while on the water.
- Close to the ocean, Tomales Bay and Drakes Estero become choppy, and high swells there can be dangerous, especially for inexperienced paddlers.
- Morning is the best time to be on the water. Winds pick up in the afternoon and may make returning to your starting point difficult and tiring.
- Be prepared for changeable weather; dress in layers and stay dry to avoid becoming chilled. Learn the signs of hypothermia and what to do should you observe them.

Etiquette on the water

- Stay at least 300 feet from wildlife; some wildlife is noticeably agitated at distances of up to 650 feet. Watch for changes in behavior, and if your presence causes a disturbance, retreat immediately.
- Do not attempt to rescue wildlife that appears sick or abandoned. Parents often leave their young alone when foraging, and you may harm the animal by interfering.
- Don't leave any trash.
- Check out www.watchablewildlife.org for their Paddler's Etiquette guidelines.

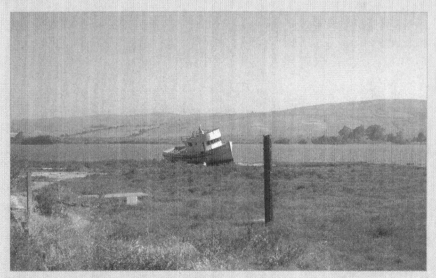

Boat on Tomales Bay marshland

accessible by car or a short trail, are described in detail in the Limantour Road, Pierce Point Road, and Palomarin trailhead sections of this book.

In Point Reyes National Seashore, Limantour and Drakes beaches on Drakes Bay are more sheltered than beaches on the open ocean. Powerful surf and a strong and unpredictable undertow make Point Reyes, Kehoe, and McClures beaches too dangerous for swimming or wading. The Pacific Ocean averages between 49 and 54°F (and is colder in summer than in winter, due to upwelling—see the section on climate).

The best swimming in the area is in Tomales Bay, at one of several sheltered beaches in **Tomales Bay State Park**. You can drive to Hearts Desire Beach, and from there walk a half mile to the more secluded Indian or Pebble beaches. At the south end of Tomales Bay State Park, a 0.3-mile path leads to Shell Beach. (See pages 207–214 for more about the park and its beaches.) No beaches in Point Reyes National Seashore or Tomales Bay State Park provide lifeguards.

Bass Lake provides the best freshwater swimming in the area. On a hot day, a dip in Bass Lake is a blissful experience. The lake is a 5.4-mile round-trip excursion from the Palomarin Trailhead. (See Trip 31.)

Five wild beaches lie between Palomarin and Limantour beaches, all accessible only by trail. These beaches are great destinations for dayhikes, and two of them are at the sites of Wildcat and Coast camps. On a backpack route up the coast, you can visit all five.

Regulations: No camping on beach, no dogs

Wildcat Beach

This 2.5-mile-long beach lies just below the scenic bluffs at Wildcat Camp. Alamere Falls cascades down the eroding cliffs at its southern end. You can count on fewer people than at more accessible beaches, since you have to hike or bike at least 5 miles to get here.

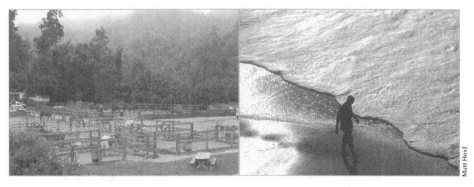

Five Brooks stables   Beach walker

Directions: Take the Coast Trail from Palomarin Trailhead or the Stewart or Greenpicker trail from Five Brooks Trailhead to reach Wildcat Beach. See Trips 27, 28, and 31 and Backpack Trips 1, 4, 6, and 7.

Facilities: Toilets, non-potable water, picnic tables at Wildcat Camp on bluff above beach

Kelham Beach

This seldom-visited beach extends for about a mile between Arch Rock and Point Resistance. A lone eucalyptus tree on the bluff above the beach marks its location and is the only remnant of Y Ranch. Nearby, a stream trickles down the cliff into the ocean.

Directions: Accessible via the Sky Trail or the Bear Valley Trail. See Trips 3 and 4 and Backpack Trip 4.

Facilities: None

Secret Beach

Secret Beach is less of a secret than it is difficult to reach. But if you time your visit to the beach with a minus tide (below 0.0 feet), you can reach Secret Beach through a passageway in the rock from neighboring Sculptured Beach. The beach itself is an isolated mile-long stretch of sand bordered by Point Resistance to the south. Several small caves and tidepools are fun to explore here.

Note: Remember that minus tides become especially high tides in a few hours. Check the tide tables before you go and keep a close eye on the tide so as not to become trapped on the beach. High, eroding cliffs prohibit climbing to the trail above.

Directions: The beach lies below the Coast Trail, just north of Kelham Beach and south of Sculptured Beach. See Trips 3, 4, 8, and 14 and Backpack Trips 4 and 5.

Facilities: None

Sculptured Beach

Wind, rain, and ocean waves have eroded the shale cliffs of Sculptured Beach to expose layers of marine sediment. Winter storms sweep away much of the sand. At low tides, you can venture southward, reaching great caves and tidepooling spots, and eventually Secret Beach, if the tide is low enough. You can also follow the beach north (across rocks or sand, depending on the season) to reach Santa Maria Beach and Coast Camp.

Directions: The beach lies below the Coast Trail, just north of Secret Beach and south of Santa Maria Beach. See Trips 3, 4, 8, and 14 and Backpack Trips 4 and 5.

Facilities: None

Santa Maria Beach

This beach lies just below Coast Camp, at the southern tip of the long stretch of Limantour Beach.

Directions: A stroll down Limantour Beach from the parking lot brings you to Santa Maria Beach in 1.5 miles. See Trips 3, 8, and 14 and Backpack Trips 1 through 5.

Facilities: Toilets, potable water, picnic tables at Coast Camp on bluff behind beach

FISHING AND CLAMMING

From Coast Miwok to the commercial fishing industry, humans have long depended on Tomales Bay for seafood and shellfish. Today, sport fishing and clamming are allowed in the bay with a California state fishing license, available through the California Department of Fish and Game (916) 227-2245 or www.dfg.ca.gov/licensing/elicense.

Lawson's Landing at the mouth of Tomales Bay is a popular spot for fishing and clamming ([707] 878-2443). Check the tides before you go, as the mudflats are revealed only at low tide. You can buy bait and tackle, clam-digging supplies, crab nets, and fishing licenses at the landing. Camping and boat launching are also available for a fee.

Herring, halibut, and leopard sharks are most commonly caught in Tomales Bay. The Department of Health and Human Services had determined that fish in Tomales Bay contain mercury contamination. It recommends strictly limiting consumption, especially for children and pregnant women, and advises against eating leopard sharks at all. Check with Marin County Environmental Health Services (415) 499-6907 or www.marin.org/ehs, or the Office of Environmental Health Hazard Assessment (916) 324-0955 www.oehha.ca.gov for details. You'll also find helpful information at www.tomalesbay.net. Note that commercially grown oysters, clams, and mussels in Tomales Bay do not contain high levels of mercury, and the health advisory does not apply to them.

PICNICKING

In the national seashore, you can drive to picnic tables at **Bear Valley headquarters**, the **Five Brooks Trailhead, Pierce Point Ranch**, and **Drakes Beach**. Hikers will find picnic tables at all **backpacking camps**. Point Reyes beaches and other sites offer opportunities for impromptu picnics. The cafe at Drakes Beach, the only food concessionaire in the park, sells clam chowder, burgers, and snacks.

Outside the seashore, you can drive to picnic sites in **Tomales Bay State Park.** On the west shore of the bay, **Hearts Desire Beach** has tables by the beach and on a bluff above the bay. (Contact the park to reserve group sites. See page 209 for more information.) On the east shore, a few picnic tables overlook **Alan Sieroty Beach.**

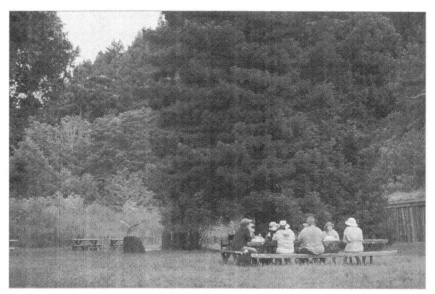
Picknickers at Bolinas Lagoon Preserve

Samuel P. Taylor State Park has picnic tables among the redwoods at the main entrance and the campgrounds. You can reserve two group picnic sites (see Samuel P. Taylor State Park, page 228). You will have a view of egrets and heron nests in the trees above the picnic tables at the **Audubon Canyon Ranch Bolinas Lagoon Preserve.**

CAMPING

The Point Reyes area offers many opportunities for overnights under the stars. **Point Reyes National Seashore** has four hike-in campgrounds, and several boat-in sites. All require an advance reservation permit. The seashore does not have any drive-in campgrounds. See pages 197–206 for details on reservations and routes in the national seashore.

Samuel P. Taylor State Park has 60 drive-to family campsites and two group camping areas. See pages 227–228 for more information. Campsites in **Tomales Bay State Park** have been closed until further notice.

Olema Ranch Campground and Lawson's Landing are two nearby private campgrounds. Farther afield, Mt. Tamalpais State Park and the Golden Gate National Recreation Area also provide camping opportunities.

WHALE-WATCHING

Every winter, Pacific gray whales travel from Alaska to the warmer waters of Baja California, where they mate and give birth before returning to Alaska. The 10,000-mile round-trip journey is one of the longest migrations of all mammals. Because they travel relatively close to shore, gray whales are easy to sight from

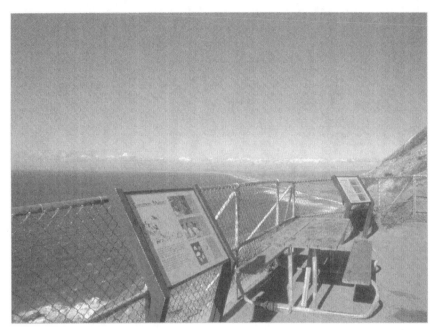
Whale lookout spot at lighthouse

coastal headlands. In December and January, pregnant females pass the Marin coast, followed by courting couples and then juveniles. In February, the whales begin the journey back north. Spring (late March to early April) is often the best time to see the migration, when mothers and their calves pass just a few hundred yards off the coast. Look for the small geysers of water that signal their presence. Lucky whale watchers will catch sight of a breaching whale—sometimes as high as 30 feet out of the water.

Jutting several miles into the ocean, **Chimney Rock** and the **lighthouse** are the best spots in the park to view whales as they make their twice-yearly migration along the coast. During the height of the migration period, sightings from the lighthouse often top 100 whales per day. Double Point (Trip 31), Millers Point (Trip 1), and other locations along the Coast Trail also provide good viewing opportunities.

Be sure to bring warm clothing and binoculars on any whale-watching excursion. For information about weather conditions and whale activity, call the Bear Valley or the Lighthouse visitor centers.

Note: On weekends and holidays from late December through mid-April, Sir Francis Drake Highway is closed at South Beach. A shuttle-bus service leaves from the Drakes Beach parking lot and takes visitors to the lighthouse and Chimney Rock. Reservations are not required. Adult tickets cost $5; children 12 and under ride free. See page 96 for more information.

Adult gray whales are about 45 feet in length—not the largest whale species by any means. But for an idea of just how big they are, the tongue alone of a gray whale weighs about 2500 pounds! Whales use their massive tongue to suck up food from the muddy ocean bottom. The food then passes through their baleen—a filter system on the roof of the mouth—before they swallow it. In the summer, whales take in about 65 tons of food in just a few months, and then feed very little during winter migration and mating.

Commercial whalers hunted gray whales for their oil almost to extinction by the early 1900s. The population has rebounded since an international hunting ban was instituted in 1946, and today numbers about 25,000, nearly as many as before they were hunted. Today, fishing nets, toxins, and noise pollution continue to threaten the health of gray whales.

Pacific gray whales aren't the only cetaceans in the Point Reyes area, just the most commonly sighted. Most other baleen whales—blue, fin, sei, minke, and beaked—rarely pass close enough to land to be seen from shore, but humpback whale sightings from Point Reyes are on the rise. If you spot a whale off the Pacific Coast in late summer or early fall, it is most likely a humpback. These acrobatic whales regularly breach and slap the water with their flippers.

Whale-watching Boat Trips

For those who want to brave the rough Pacific waters to get a closer look at whales, the Oceanic Society (415-474-3385) and Bodega Bay Fishing (707-875-3495) offer expeditions by boat.

BIRDING

Point Reyes is a birdwatcher's paradise. Birders flock here to glimpse some of the nearly 490 species that live in or pass through this area each year. In addition to the abundance of bird species who are "regulars" at Point Reyes, the peninsula attracts a large number of "vagrants" who wander off their normal migratory path and end up on the peninsula.

Most anywhere you visit in the Point Reyes area, you're likely to see a remarkable number of birds—acorn woodpeckers in the picnic area at Bear Valley, hawks perched on fences and telephone poles along the road, and herons in the tidal flats along Tomales Bay. The following are a few especially good places to look for birds.

Good Birding Spots

Most birders head first to the **outer point**, the vicinity of vagrants and seabirds. In the fall, join the groups of birders looking for vagrant warblers in the cypress trees near A and B ranches. The cliffs and offshore rocks near the **lighthouse** are home to many seabirds, including Brandt's cormorants, common murres, and brown pelicans. At **Chimney Rock**, loons, grebes, and harlequin ducks gather near the fish docks in Drakes Bay. Take the trail to the tip of Chimney Rock to see peregrine falcons, cormorants, common murres, and pelicans. Great-horned owls often nest in the cypress trees near the Drake monument at **Drakes Beach**. Look for long-eared and barn owl roosts in Monterey pines along the Estero Trail at **Drakes Estero**, about a half mile from the trailhead. Farther along the trail, you're likely to see herons, egrets, and godwits in the estero, and brown and white pelicans near the coast. At the northern reaches of the outer point, numerous shorebirds visit **Abbotts Lagoon**. Look for grebes, ruddy ducks, kites, and white pelicans, especially during fall and winter. Snowy plovers nest in the dunes near the lagoon during spring and summer.

In the Limantour area, the **Bayview Trail** near Muddy Hollow attracts Wilson's warblers, black-headed grosbeaks, wrens, bushtits, and various flycatchers. The trail along **Limantour Spit** provides great opportunities to see the fall shorebird migration and waterfowl in winter.

Bear Valley is a good place to watch the spring migration of many landbird species, especially in riparian areas along Olema Creek and on the Bear Valley and Earthquake trails. In winter, climb to the top of Mt. Wittenberg on the Sky Trail to look for bluebirds. Walk the Bear Valley Trail in May, listening for the distinctive, piercing call of the osprey. From their nests high in the Douglas-firs

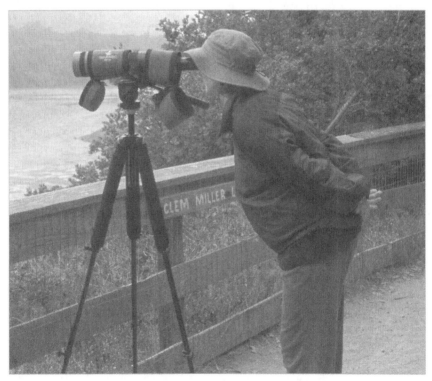

Looking at heron and egret nests at Bolinas Lagoon Preserve

on Inverness Ridge, these fish-eating birds fly to the ocean, Tomales Bay, Nicasio Reservoir and Bolinas Lagoon to find food for themselves and their young.

Freshwater **Olema Marsh** attracts waterbirds, herons, swallows, and finches, as well as fall migrants like thrushes, warblers, and sparrows. You'll almost always see kites at the marsh. **Five Brooks Pond** is a good place to see migratory birds, especially between August and October, in the riparian willows and alders. Look for wood ducks and grebes in the pond.

Several species of shorebirds feed at **Bolinas Lagoon**, including great blue herons and great and snowy egrets that nest at the **Audubon Canyon Ranch Bolinas Lagoon Preserve**, just east of the lagoon. Visit the preserve in spring for an up-close view of their nests and chicks through spotting scopes provided at the viewing overlook. **Pine Gulch Creek** empties into the lagoon on its west side, and its dense riparian vegetation is often full of birds. At the **Point Reyes Bird Observatory** (PRBO), you'll likely see wrentits, white-crowned sparrows, towhees, and Wilson's warblers, among many others. The visitor center at PBRO is an extraordinary place to see and learn about birds. PRBO naturalists also offer guided walks every month, as well as classes.

You can participate in a Point Reyes National Seashore Association Field Seminar to learn more about birds in the Point Reyes area. Local birding experts give one-day and weekend courses on everything from owls, to fall and spring migrants, to bird calls.

Note: Many ranches on the peninsula are still active operations and residences. Birders are welcome to cross ranch lands, but should be respectful of the property and animals, and park away from the farm buildings, not blocking any gates.

TIDEPOOLING

Many Point Reyes beaches provide great opportunities for tidepooling. A fascinating array of invertebrates and algae inhabit the intertidal community— between low and high tide marks. These unique organisms can survive both immersion in ocean water and exposure to air.

Tidepooling Tips

Before you go, check the tide tables to find low tide times. Point Reyes beaches are often windy and foggy, so dress warmly. Wear shoes that you don't mind getting wet and that provide good traction. Be careful where you step—the rocks in the intertidal zone are often "alive" with plant and animal life. Keep your eye on the water for unexpected waves and always be aware of the tide schedule— some beaches are inaccessible at high tide, and you could easily become trapped.

Good Tidepooling Beaches

Palomarin, Kehoe, McClures, Sculptured

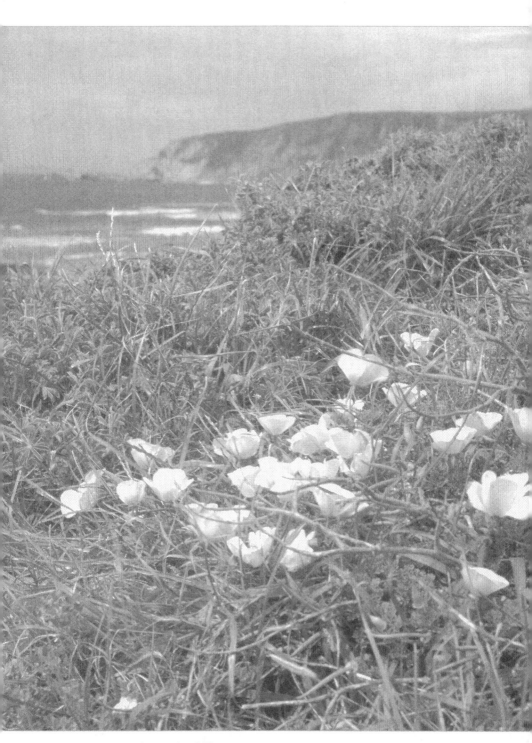

Kehoe with wildflowers

WILDFLOWER VIEWING

In spring, almost any trail in Point Reyes National Seashore rewards hikers and walkers with a colorful display of wildflowers, from milkmaids and hound's-tongues in forests to buttercups, iris, and suncups in grasslands. A few places put on extra-special spring shows. **Chimney Rock** always tops "Best wildflower spots" lists and is well-deserving of the ranking, as the coastal grasslands and cliffs dance with color in spring. Keep an eye out for two special flowers in the lily family that appear at Chimney Rock: the fuzzy, lavender petals of pussy ears (*Calochortus tolmiei*) and the nodding, mottled flowers of mission bells (*Fritillaria lanceolata*). **Abbotts Lagoon** is another exceptional wildflower spot, where brilliant swaths of goldfields and numerous other species cover the hillsides. Baby blue eyes, poppies, and more paint the bluffs behind **Kehoe Beach,** and the **Coast, Bayview,** and **Tomales Point trails** all provide excellent wildflower displays.

East of the peninsula, suncups, flax, blue-eyed grass, buttercups, and other grasslands wildflowers bloom along the **Tomales Bay, Millerton Point,** and **Bolinas Ridge trails** (on GGNRA and Tomales Bay State Park land).

TOURING THE POINT REYES AREA

In addition to the multitude of recreation and nature activities at Point Reyes, the area has a flourishing cultural life and an active agricultural economy. Art galleries, bookstores, farmers' markets, and eateries round out a day at the seashore or one of the nearby parks, or fill a weekend of just poking around. You'll find fun activities, good food, and a glimpse into the intriguing history of West Marin.

POINT REYES TOWNS
Highway 1, South to North

The town of **Bolinas** lies at the southern end of the Olema Valley, between the Bolinas Lagoon and the flat mesa at the tip of the Point Reyes peninsula that stretches to the Pacific Coast. After repeatedly removing the sign to Bolinas on Highway 1, residents finally succeeded in achieving permanent unsigned status. (Go west on the road at the north end of Bolinas Lagoon; bear left again at the junction with Mesa Road and continue to town.) The town's central area is composed of two streets—one that terminates at the coast and the other at the lagoon—and is best visited on foot. Known for a lively art scene, Bolinas has several shops and galleries, and the **Bolinas Museum** (48 Wharf Road, 415-868-0330) hosts local and historic art exhibits. The community center offers classes, concerts, and films. You'll also find a market, a natural foods store, and several cafes and restaurants, as well as essential services like a laundromat, gas station, and medical clinic.

Has a brief visit to Point Reyes piqued your interest in the park and its ecosystems? Have its birds, flowers, tidepools, beaches, and history instilled an awe of the peninsula? Are you ready to learn more about Point Reyes National Seashore? Here are a few ways you can get to know Point Reyes better:

Educational Resources

The National Park Service and the **Point Reyes National Seashore Association (PRNSA)** offer fun and interesting educational opportunities for all ages. **PRNSA Field Seminars,** taught by well-known professionals, include one- or two-day classes about natural history—bird songs, spring and fall migrant birds, owls and hawks, wildflowers, mosses and lichens, and native shrubs—and art—basket making, sketching, photography, and water coloring.

Kids who join the **Junior Ranger program** (ages 5 to 12) receive their own park ranger badge and certificate. Two summer camps for kids, **Nature Science Camp and Adventure Camp**, offer tidepooling, birding, boating, and camping adventures.

The **Point Reyes Bird Observatory (PRBO)** offers free bird walks, lectures and presentations for groups, and resources for schoolteachers and classes. See the section in this book on PRBO for more information about visiting the bird observatory.

Volunteer Opportunities

The **National Park Service** recruits docents for snowy plover and tule elk programs. **PRNSA** welcomes volunteers to do office work and to staff seminars,

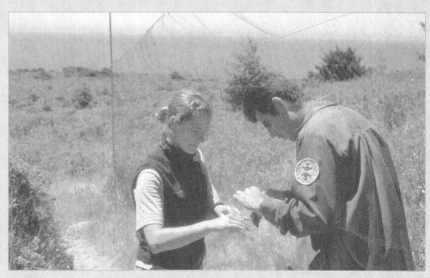

Interns at Point Reyes Bird Observatory

hikes, and events. Contact the organization for more information about how you can participate as a volunteer. At **Audubon Canyon Ranch Bolinas Lagoon Preserve,** volunteers can work as docents and guides, and help out with habitat restoration. See pages 221–224 for more information.

For Teachers and Students

The **Clem Miller Environmental Education Center** hosts teachers and their students for 3 or 5 days; the center provides training and teaching materials to teachers, who lead their own programs. The Point Reyes National Seashore website has details about how the center is run, what it provides, and how to make reservations (www.nps.gov/pore).

Park rangers and resources specialists teach workshops for teachers who want to bring their classes to Point Reyes. Workshops provide training, curricula materials, and tips on visiting the park with school groups.

Ranger-led programs for schoolchildren take classes to the lighthouse and Kule Loklo, the replica Coast Miwok village, or teach them about park wildlife and history.

The Point Reyes Bird Observatory offers many resources for schoolteachers and their classes. Call them or visit their website for more details. (www.prbo.org)

The Pacific Coast Learning Center

More than a recreation area, Point Reyes National Seashore is also a dynamic, hands-on research environment for scientists, researchers, and students. The National Park Service established the Pacific Coast Learning Center to encourage research about park resources; it provides financial support, laboratory and computer facilities, and housing. Research about spotted owls, snowy plovers, fish biodiversity in Tomales Bay, subtidal habitats, and more help the park make informed decisions about managing natural resources. For more information, see www.nps.gov/pore/science.htm or contact the park.

Point Reyes National Seashore Association

PRNSA, founded in 1964, works with the National Park Service to preserve and protect the park's natural and cultural resources by providing resources and funding for park projects and programs. PRNSA has helped create interpretive displays at the visitor centers and at Kule Loklo, construct the Clem Miller Environmental Education Center, publish books including *The Natural History of Point Reyes,* by Jules Evens, and *Coast Miwok Indians of Point Reyes,* by Sylvia Thalman. Field Seminars, an Elderhostel program, and a Science and Adventure Camp for kids help visitors of all ages learn about Point Reyes National Seashore. The association is also involved with projects like native plant restoration, snowy plover protection and monitoring, and habitat restoration in the Vision Fire area.

The route to the Palomarin Trailhead in Point Reyes National Seashore skirts Bolinas and passes the Point Reyes Bird Observatory (PRBO). PRBO and Audubon Canyon Ranch Bolinas Lagoon Preserve (east of the lagoon) are excellent spots for birding and short hikes (see Birding section, pages 75–77).

From Bolinas, go north on Highway 1 to reach the town of **Olema**. Visitors approaching Point Reyes from the east on Sir Francis Drake Highway will look down into the furrow of the Olema Valley from the crest of Bolinas Ridge and then dip into the valley to arrive at Olema, the closest town to park headquarters at Bear Valley.

Although small, Olema keeps several shops, restaurants, and inns in business due to its crossroads location and its proximity to seashore headquarters. Today, two popular restaurants, the **Olema Farmhouse** (built in 1845—the oldest building in town, 415-663-1264) and the **Olema Inn and Restaurant** (which dates back to 1876, 415-663-9559), serve local specials in historic buildings. In the late 1800s, the town was the lively hub of West Marin, known for its six bars. A biweekly stagecoach service traveled to San Rafael and a schooner service ran to San Francisco from the foot of Tomales Bay, 2 miles away.

Two miles north of Olema on Highway 1, you reach **Point Reyes Station.** Bustling with activity on weekends, Point Reyes Station is a quiet community during the week, with a mixture of stores and restaurants that cater to locals— ranchers, shopkeepers, weekenders, park employees—and tourists. First known as Olema Station, the town grew up when the North Pacific Coast Railroad reached West Marin in 1875 and established a depot in what was then a cow pasture. Over the next few years, the town burgeoned with several shops and residences, a school, and a post office. In 1882 the name was officially changed to Point Reyes Station.

Pick up a copy of the *Point Reyes Light*, the town's weekly newspaper, to find news and events for Point Reyes Station and vicinity. The *Light* won a Pulitzer Prize (one of few weekly newspapers ever to do so) for its 1979 exposé of the Synanon cult scandal, which took place just up the road at what is now the Marconi Conference Center. Point Reyes Station's community center, the Dance Palace, is a thriving cultural hub for West Marin. Jazz concerts, choral groups, contemporary music, plays, films, and art exhibits are among the events you'll find at the center, along with yoga, ceramics, art, and aikido classes for kids and adults. Check the listings in the *Point Reyes Light* or the website at www.dancepalace.org or call (415) 663-1075 for events and classes.

KWMR 90.5 FM, broadcast from the historic Creamery Building in Point Reyes Station, provides information about the local scene and an array of entertainment. Local deejays play world and classical music and host current events discussions and author talks.

For a sampling of local artists' work, stop by **Gallery Route One** (415-663-1347), where exhibitions by professional artists explore cultural, political, and environmental concerns. Up the street, visit the **Marty Knapp Photography** gallery (415-663-8670) to see his hand-printed black and white photos that capture the dramatic Point Reyes landscape. In the next block, the **Point Reyes Bookstore** (415-663-1542) has an excellent collection of new and used books, and hosts frequent readings and events with authors from near and far. Check their schedule for cooking demonstrations with cookbook authors, Spanish conversation groups, benefits for local libraries, and more.

Next door, a line stretches out the door of the **Bovine Bakery**, where you can stop for scrumptious scones, muffins, or pastries; pizzas and soups; and cookies, pies, and brownies. The bakery also sells organic **Brickmaiden Bread**, made just a few doors away. Across the street, you'll find the basics at the **Palace Market**; look for local specialty foods at the **Cowgirl Creamery** and the **Indian Peach Food Company** around the corner in **Tomales Bay Foods** (see section on local food). Several restaurants offer good options for sit-down meals. **The Station House Cafe** has been in town since 1974, serving local mussels and oysters plus salads, burgers, and vegetarian dishes. Open for breakfast, lunch, and dinner (415) 663-1515.

Tomales Bay West Shore
Sir Francis Drake Highway heads west from Highway 1 just south of Point Reyes Station. The road bisects freshwater Olema Marsh, where alders, willows, tule, and cattails provide an ideal habitat for birds, and then heads up the west shore of Tomales Bay, en route to the lighthouse, Pierce Point, Drakes Estero, Tomales Bay State Park, and northern beaches. Steep side roads periodically

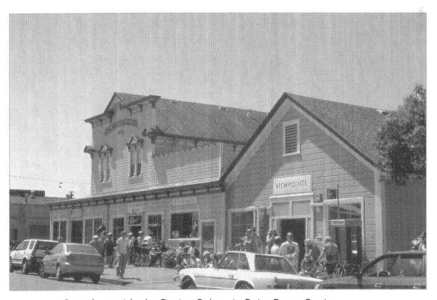

Crowds outside the Bovine Bakery in Point Reyes Station

leave the two-lane highway to climb to homes on the tree-covered slopes of Inverness Ridge.

You soon reach the small communities of **Inverness Park** and **Inverness**. Both towns have a general store and deli, and an abundance of inns and B&Bs (see Lodging section). **Debra's Bakery** whips up treats in Inverness Park, and in Inverness, **Manka's Inverness Lodge** serves acclaimed meals, using local ingredients like wild mushrooms, huckleberries, fish, game, and rabbit. Several stores in both communities sell arts and crafts.

The slopes of Inverness Ridge on the west shore of Tomales Bay are home to several artists whom you can visit during Point Reyes Open Studios (see page 88) or by appointment. Printmaker Rick Lyttle creates local landscapes and whimsical scenes using mezzotint, aquatint, etching, and lithography, among other printing techniques. Call ahead to visit his studio (415-663-1457); with a few days advance notice, he'll demonstrate his printmaking and pull a print on

LANDSCAPE PAINTER SUSAN HALL

"What makes us human is our connection to the land."

The simple, striking landscapes that painter Susan Hall renders reflect a lifetime at Point Reyes. Born during World War II, Susan Hall grew up in Point Reyes Station when it was still a distant outpost from the bustling city. Kids spent slow Sunday afternoons counting passing cars from the corner gas station—and usually tallied only five or six.

Susan remembers the peninsula as it was before the park was established, when most residents were ranch families or employees of AT&T and RCA, like her father. "You could feel the wildness," she says. Even as a young girl, she knew the richness of Point Reyes: "I never took a day of my life for granted growing up here."

At an early age, Susan Hall also knew her future as a painter. A long and fruitful art career has led her back to the landscapes of home. As she says, she paints memories: her memories create tangible layers of time and relationships—they enliven and complete the landscape. The light and hills and bay and cliffs and ocean and trees in her paintings resonate with accumulated years of seeing and with the memories each seeing triggers.

Few people know Point Reyes as intimately as Susan Hall does; of the 2.5 million visitors who come to Point Reyes National Seashore each year, most are transient. She hopes that through her art she can help people know this place and get them to "dive deeper." Susan Hall understands the importance of the human presence in the Point Reyes landscape; she wants "tourists to see how people lived here in modest ways that fit into the environment."

his impressive Allen Gregg press. Four guest artists use the press, including Gary Smith and Nancy Stein, whose work you can view in their own studios during Point Reyes Open Studios. The California coast and the High Sierra are the subjects of Tom Killion's woodcut and linocut prints. You can make an appointment to visit his Inverness studio (415-663-1516) or view his work at one of his spring or fall art shows.

Point Reyes landowner James Shafter, crushed by heavy losses in railroad investments, founded the town of Inverness in an attempt to recover the family fortune. He created hundreds of lots along Tomales Bay and sold them to wealthy San Franciscans for weekend homes. The city folk arrived by train at Point Reyes Station and rode the remaining four miles to Inverness by stage.

On Park Way in Inverness, just off of Sir Francis Drake, the **Jack Mason Museum** houses the late historian Jack Mason's extensive collection of photos, books, manuscripts, and artifacts of West Marin history. The author of several

Her paintings both embrace your own experience of the landscape and invite you to step beyond yourself and know the land on a deeper level. They unite what you know and what you might only sense.

Susan Hall participates in the Point Reyes Open Studios, held on Thanksgiving and Fourth of July weekends, and in MALT's *Ranches and Rolling Hills* landscape art show and sale. She has published a collection of her work in her book *Painting Point Reyes*. You can also see some of her art at www.susan-hall.org.

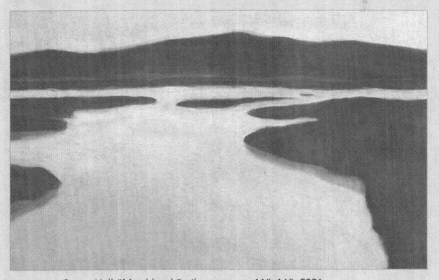

Susan Hall "Marshland," oil on canvas, 11"x16", 2001

books on local history, Jack Mason willed his charming Victorian house to serve as a museum and as the **Inverness Public Library**. For visiting hours, call (415) 669-1099.

About 4 miles past Inverness, you reach the Golden Hinde Inn and Marina and, just beyond, Blue Waters Kayaking, where you can rent or launch kayaks.

Tomales Bay East Shore

From Point Reyes Station, a scenic drive north along the east shore of Tomales Bay takes you to **Millerton Point** and Alan Sieroty Beach (see Tomales Bay State Park, pages 207–214). Just beyond, you reach the **Tomales Bay Oyster Company,** one of several oyster farms in the area where you can buy fresh oysters to barbeque on-site or take home for a delicious dinner (see Local Food, below).

A few miles farther north, you pass the **Marconi Conference Center**, on the east side of the highway, also a state historic park (415-663-9020). The center has a colorful history, first as a radio receiving station built by Guglielmo Marconi (the inventor of the wireless telegraph) and much later, in the 1970s, as home base for the Synanon cult. Up the road at **Tamal Saka Kayaks** you can rent a boat to explore Tomales Bay.

The town of **Marshall** is just beyond, perhaps best known today for the oysters that are grown in offshore tidal beds. The working oyster farm **Hog Island Oyster Company** sells oysters and clams. Bring a picnic and enjoy the view from waterfront tables (see Local Food, below).

Two brothers from Ireland founded Marshall in the 1850s, and they had established a bustling settlement even before the railroad came through on its

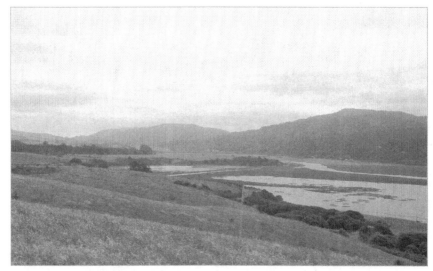

Looking south along Tomales Bay's east shore

way to North Coast redwoods in 1875. Following the area's long tradition of dairy farming, the **Straus Family Creamery** operates in the hills east of town (not open to the public). Continuing north on Highway 1, about a half mile past the Marshall–Petaluma Road, the buildings of the Audubon Canyon Ranch **Cypress Grove Preserve** are mostly hidden from view, on the west side of the road. The preserve functions as a research center and is not open to the public (see page 224).

A few miles beyond, at **Miller County Park**, you can use the fishing pier, boat launching facilities, and picnic tables for a small entrance fee (toilets available).

Highway 1 continues north along the shore of Tomales Bay and heads inland at the marshy mouth of Walker and Keys creeks. Look for egrets and other shorebirds among the rushes. The highway shortly reaches the small town of **Tomales**, where you can snack on fresh breads and pastries from the Tomales Bakery while surveying the low-key hum of the town from its outdoor patio.

The **Tomales Regional History Center** depicts the boisterous railroad town that Tomales once was—several bars, a bowling alley, and a horse race track provided local entertainment. The center is housed in the auditorium of the old high school, at the south end of town (Open 1 to 4 P.M., Friday through Sunday or by appointment, 707-878-9443.)

Check the back page of the *Point Reyes Light* for the "Guide to the Coast," featuring listings of restaurants, lodging, galleries, and outings in the area. Also pick up the free *Coastal Traveler*, issued quarterly by the *Point Reyes Light* and available in most businesses in West Marin, for up-to-date information on restaurants, lodgings, stores, and activities from Marin north to Mendocino and Lake counties.

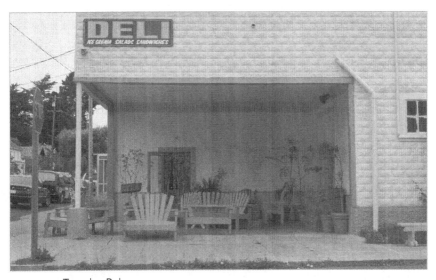

Tomales Bakery

Point Reyes Open Studios

Twice a year, Point Reyes artists open their home studios to the public, revealing art inspired by the Point Reyes landscape. Over Fourth of July and Thanksgiving weekends, nearly two dozen artists in Point Reyes Station, Inverness, and Olema show their work, from paintings and etchings to ceramics, textiles, and photographs.

To find out more about Point Reyes Open Studios and about local artists and their work, check out www.pointreyesart.com.

LOCAL FOOD AND AGRICULTURE

Cows in a national park? Some people are surprised to see bovines on pasturelands in Point Reyes National Seashore—others are thrilled. Either way, most people are curious. Agriculture has a long history at Point Reyes and still flourishes on the rolling grasslands and tranquil bays within the national seashore and in the surrounding area. Long before it was a park, Point Reyes supported one of the largest dairy industries in California. Today, six dairy ranches, nine beef cattle ranches, and one oyster farm operate within Point Reyes National Seashore; numerous ranches and farms raise animals and grow crops in and around Tomales Bay.

Some of these small businesses have been in operation for over a century, run by the same families for generations; others are more recent arrivals to West Marin. Both long-time ranchers and innovative newcomers are embracing a growing movement toward local food production and natural or organic products. Much of the meat, dairy products, vegetables, and seafood from these ranches and farms aren't shipped to distant consumers: they go directly to nearby restaurants and stores or become the ingredients for locally produced specialty products.

They are also the ingredients for a healthy rural landscape and economy. While groups like the Marin Agricultural Land Trust work with ranchers to save their land from development and to preserve agriculture, this region's rural heritage won't continue unless it is economically and environmentally viable. So far, several Point Reyes farms have proven that a niche in the market of locally produced specialty foods is viable. Local cheese, wine, milk, butter, oysters, and olive oil have all won prestigious national awards, and the market—in the San Francisco Bay Area and nationally—has embraced these products with enthusiasm.

As you tour the Point Reyes area, you'll pass grazing cattle and sheep, fields of organic produce, olive groves, rows of grapevines, and oyster beds. Within the seashore, signs along the road mark historic ranches, and you'll see working dairies as you rumble over cattle guards on your way to trailheads and beaches. **Murphy Ranch** rears all-natural beef on the historic Home Ranch site near

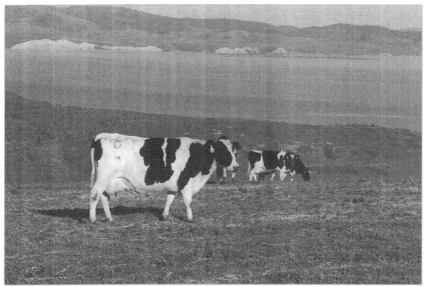
Point Reyes cows

Drakes Estero, sharing the pasture with deer, rabbits, and birds. **Johnson's Oyster Company**, the only remaining commercial enterprise on Drakes Estero, is near the site of the old schooner landing where butter—the original Point Reyes product—was shipped to San Francisco. On the peninsula's northern tip, the family that runs **Marin Sun Farms** has grazed cows on the rich grasslands for four generations. The farm now raises grass-fed beef and free-range chickens.

En route to the Palomarin Trailhead and the Point Reyes Bird Observatory, you'll pass **Niman Ranch** cows on the coastal mesa. The all-natural meat goes from these hillsides to the plates of some of the Bay Area's best restaurants. Nearby, **Star Route Farms** grows lettuce, leeks, and baby carrots. A pioneer in the organic movement in California, the farm has cultivated specialty greens and vegetables in Bolinas since the early 1970s, and sends their produce to some of the most prestigious restaurants around. Star Route Farms and other growers around Bolinas have worked with the National Park Service to balance agricultural water needs with the water requirements of the fish that spawn in nearby creeks. (See Coho Salmon and Steelhead Trout Restoration, pages 36–38.)

The east side of Tomales Bay is also replete with agricultural riches. As Highway 1 crests a small rise north of Point Reyes Station, you look down on a tapestry of grapevines on the hillside behind **Point Reyes Vineyard Inn**. In this unique combination of dairy farm, vineyard, and bed and breakfast, this long-time Point Reyes family has combined tradition and innovation. (You can visit the tasting room on Saturdays and Sundays between 9 A.M. and 5 P.M.) Just beyond, you'll pass the sign for **Giacomini Dairy**, where the family grazes cows for milk and cheese (not open to the public; see page 93).

Farther north along the scenic route, you can take a short walk along the bluff at Millerton Point and look out over oyster beds in Tomales Bay, where the shellfish delicacies grow from seed. The **Straus Family Creamery** is tucked in the folds of the hills above Marshall. Its cows grazing these hillsides produce organic milk, yogurt, cheese, ice cream, and butter. (You can visit many of these ranches on Marin Agricultural Land Trust tours. See pages 52–53 for more information.)

Sampling Local Food Products

Your stomach grumbling, your mouth watering, and nearby trails and beaches beckoning with perfect picnic spots, stop by a local market to sample some of these tasty local products. In Point Reyes Station, **Tomales Bay Foods** buzzes with activity as both a showcase for the agricultural riches of Point Reyes and a gathering place for local ranchers and farmers. The renovated hay barn houses the **Cowgirl Creamery** in one corner, which makes cheese behind glass walls and sells it a few steps away. **Goldenpoint Produce** sells fruit and vegetables from local farms. **Indian Peach Food Company**, a take-away restaurant, makes soups, salads, sandwiches, entrees, and desserts, mostly from local and organic produce and meat. Pick up a loaf of bread made next door and complete your picnic with a bottle of local wine. (Open Wednesday through Sunday, 10 A.M. to 6 P.M. On B Street between 3rd and 4th, one block west of Highway 1.)

Just down the street from Tomales Bay Foods, **Toby's Feed Barn** provides hay and feed for ranchers, as well as the end products for consumers. Vendors at a weekly **farmers' market** in front sell local vegetables, flowers, olive oil, and jams. (Open 9 A.M. to 5 P.M., Monday through Saturday; 9:30 to 4:30, Sunday;

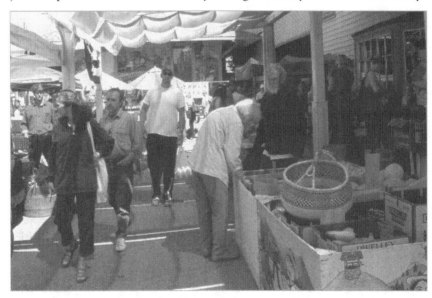

Farmers' market

farmers' market 9 A.M. to 1 P.M., Saturdays in summer. On Highway 1 in the center of town.)

At **Hog Island Oyster Company** you can feast on fresh oysters and manila clams at waterfront picnic tables. The farm (not a restaurant) provides shucking knives and barbeque kettles; you bring the picnic. (Open 9 A.M. to 5 P.M., Wednesday through Sunday. On Highway 1 in Marshall.) **Tomales Bay Oyster Company** also sells oysters to the public and provides tables and barbeques. (Open 8 A.M. to 6 P.M., every day. On Highway 1 about 5 miles north of Point Reyes Station.)

At **Johnson's Oyster Company**, see if you can taste the difference between oysters grown in Tomales Bay and those from the waters of Drakes Estero. (Open 8:30 A.M. to 4:30 P.M., Tuesday through Friday; 9:30 A.M. to 4:30 P.M., Saturday and Sunday. From Sir Francis Drake Highway, turn left on a road signed to the oyster company.)

Johnson's grows, harvests and sells fresh Pacific oysters in three sizes. While Drakes Estero is too cold for oysters to spawn naturally, it does allow them to be harvested year-round. Spawning takes place in a lab where millions of microscopic larvae and water are added to tanks filled with old oyster shells. After the larvae attach or set themselves on shells, bags of the shells are hung in the bay for about two months. After this initial period of growth, the shells are strung to 8-foot-long wires and returned to the water where they remain for another 18 to 24 months. Suspended above the bottom mud, the maturing oysters are protected from predators such as crabs and sea stars.

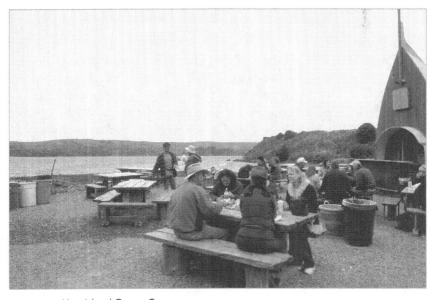

Hog Island Oyster Company

Creamy rounds of organic cheese and crumbly chunks of tangy blue cheese are some of Point Reyes' delicious local products, but cheesemaking is nothing new to this area. In fact, the renowned Point Reyes dairy industry of the 1800s, celebrated for its butter, began with a recipe for cheese and an entrepreneurial rancher's wife. With stagecoach, schooner, and train as the only means of transportation, the journey from Point Reyes to city markets was too far for unrefrigerated milk. So Point Reyes dairies turned milk into cheese and butter—and created a thriving dairy industry widely known for the quality of its products. When transportation improved, these dairies began to sell milk and gave up butter and cheese production. Today, Point Reyes dairies have come full circle: as milk prices decrease, dairy ranchers looking for a financially sustainable way to remain on the family farm are finding a viable niche market in value-added products like cheese and other locally produced food. The dairy industry at Point Reyes is once again wowing city folk with the quality of its cheese.

The "terroir" of Point Reyes—its unique climate and premier pastureland—is key to the flavor of local cheese. In the 19th century, aficionados explained the exceptional quality of Point Reyes dairy products by the long growing season and the fresh green grass. Cheesemakers today still attribute the exceptional flavors of their cheeses to the salty ocean air, temperature, moisture, and grasses here. Even just 30 miles away, a different combination of soil and microclimate would lend a different flavor to the cheese. Fog rolls in with early morning and afternoon breezes, nurturing the sweet grasses, creating a long growing season, and keeping the humidity high—a perfect environment for the creamy texture and rich taste of these cheeses.

Cowgirl Creamery

The Cowgirl Creamery in Point Reyes Station makes cheese the traditional way—by hand, in small batches, and without additives. Their mission, as much as it is to make good cheese, is to support local dairies and sustainable agriculture. They make all their cheese with organic milk from the Straus Family Creamery, just up the road in Marshall. The Straus dairy, in operation since 1941, has found its niche as an organic dairy; in addition to the milk they sell to Cowgirl Creamery, Straus sells organic milk, yogurt, butter, ice cream, and a few of their own cheeses nationwide.

Cowgirl Creamery produces about 300 pounds of cheese a week, including an old-fashioned cottage cheese, a light and flavorful fromage blanc, and a rich crème fraiche. Their small rounds of triple-cream and whole-milk cheese go by names like Mt. Tam, Red Hawk, and Pierce Point. The creamery commemorates the arrival of spring with St. Pat, a whole-milk cheese wrapped in the leaves of stinging nettles that grow nearby (washed and frozen to get rid of the sting).

The cowgirls' hard work has been rewarded by an enthusiastic reception from individuals and well-known Bay Area restaurants. Tomales Bay Foods, the gourmet market Cowgirl Creamery founders opened in Point Reyes Station, does a brisk business in their own cheeses, as well as cheeses from Europe and other parts of the United States. You can watch the cheesemakers at work Wednesday through Sunday, between 10 A.M. and 6 P.M. Then visit the cheese counter and see if you can taste the terroir of Point Reyes. Check out their website at www.cowgirlcreamery.com.

Point Reyes Farmstead Cheese Company

Nearby, Point Reyes cows are milked for another locally produced cheese. The Giacomini family, long-time Point Reyes dairy ranchers but newcomers to the cheese business, make the only farmstead blue cheese in California ("farmstead" means the ingredients come exclusively from the farm where the product is made). Bob Giacomini has been raising cows for milk on his farm above Tomales Bay since 1959; before that, his grandfather and father raised chickens and dairy cows in Petaluma and Point Reyes.

But dairying is no easy business, especially for a small dairy on environmentally sensitive land. After realizing that runoff from dairies around Tomales Bay contributes to pollution in the waters, Mr. Giacomini began to look for a way to reduce his herd of 500 cows and still remain economically viable. He also wanted to entice his daughters, who had left for careers in the city, to return to the farm.

The Giacominis combined their dairying experience with marketing savvy and found a new direction for the dairy—one that brought the family back to the area and met the growing interest in locally produced food: the Giacominis decided to enter the cheese market. Before deciding what kind of cheese to produce, they approached local chefs to find out where there was a gap in the market. Chefs immediately responded with "blue cheese." So the family dairy became the Point Reyes Farmstead Cheese Company. They converted the horse barn to a cheese plant, reduced their herd of cows to about 250, retrained their employees to manufacturing positions, and lured a master blue-cheese maker from Iowa to their ranch.

Point Reyes Farmstead makes cheese four days a week; the other three, the dairy continues to sell milk to processing plants. The farmstead cheese has succeeded in economically sustaining the family farm, in bringing the family back to the business, and in reducing at least one farm's impact on the health of the ecosystem.

You can learn more about the company and their cheese on their website at www.pointreyescheese.com.

LODGING

You'll find plenty of lodging options in the Point Reyes area—from inns, B&Bs, and cottages to vacation rentals, hotels, and motels—with a variety of views, styles, locations, and prices. For complete listings and assistance, contact one of the free lodging services in the area or the West Marin Chamber of Commerce.

Point Reyes Hostel

Tucked in a protected coastal valley, the Point Reyes hostel offers lodging for families, groups, and individuals—young and old alike—and is the only lodging within the national seashore other than camping. Run by Hosteling International, the facility is wheelchair-accessible and provides a self-service kitchen, 44 beds and one private room (reserved for families with children age five or younger), and on-site parking. Visitors must be gone from the premises between 10:00 A.M. and 4:30 P.M. Check-in time is between 4:30 and 9:30 P.M.. To make a reservation (recommended, with a MasterCard or Visa), call between 7:30 and 9:30 A.M. or 4:30 and 9:30 P.M..

Phone: (415) 663-8811. **Rates:** $22 per night

Driving Directions: From the Bear Valley Visitor Center, return to Bear Valley Road. Turn left and drive 1.5 miles to Limantour Road. Turn left again, follow the road for 6 miles and turn left onto Laguna Road. The hostel is on your left 0.2 mile beyond.

Inns of Marin

Point Reyes, CA 94956
(415) 663-2000, Fax (415) 669-7424, E-mail: julie@innsofmarin.com

Point Reyes Lodging

P.O. Box 878
Point Reyes Station, CA 94956
(415) 663-1872, (800) 539-1872, www.ptreyes.com

West Marin Network

11434 Shoreline Highway, Old Creamery Building, Suite 17
Point Reyes Station, CA 94956
(415) 663-9543, Fax (415) 663-8275

West Marin Chamber of Commerce

P.O. Box 1045, Point Reyes Station, CA 94956
(415) 663-9232, E-mail: info@pointreyes.org

Opposite page: Double Point

Point Reyes Trails and Beaches

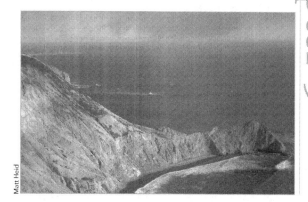

Chapter 5

Matt Heid

VISITOR INFORMATION

DIRECTIONS TO POINT REYES

These directions take you to park headquarters at Bear Valley, from the towns of Olema and Point Reyes Station. For directions to these towns see page 55 in Chapter 4.

From the junction of Sir Francis Drake Highway and Highway 1 in Olema, make an immediate left on Bear Valley Rd. Continue 0.5 mile to the visitor center road; turn left and go 0.2 mile to a large paved parking area.

From Point Reyes Station, follow Highway 1 through town and just after crossing the green bridge, turn right on Sir Francis Drake Blvd. Go 0.7 mile to Bear Valley Rd., turn left, and continue 1.7 miles to the visitor center road. Turn right and go 0.2 mile to a large paved parking area.

West Marin roads are narrow and winding. Numerous bicyclists and motorcyclists tour these roads, especially on weekends. Please drive with extreme caution, pass only in legally designated sections and when you are certain all is clear, and use turnouts when necessary.

During heavy storms, some West Marin roads may be closed due to flooding or fallen trees. Call Caltrans at (800) 427-7623 or (415) 557-3755.

Getting there by bus:

Golden Gate Transit
(415) 923-2000

Bus #63 goes from Marin City to Audubon Canyon Ranch Bolinas Lagoon Preserve on weekends while the preserve is open.

West Marin Stagecoach
(415)526-3239, www.marin-stagecoach.org

Weekday service from San Anselmo to Samuel P. Taylor State Park, Olema, Point Reyes Station, and Inverness; from Marin City to Muir Beach, Stinson Beach, and Bolinas.

TRANSPORTATION WITHIN THE PARK

From park headquarters at Bear Valley, you will need a car to reach all trailheads other than Bear Valley.

On weekends and holidays from late-December to mid-April (prime whale-watching and wildflower-viewing season) the park closes Sir Francis Drake Highway at South Beach and runs a shuttle-bus service from Drakes Beach to the lighthouse and Chimney Rock. You can purchase tickets at the Ken Patrick Visitor Center at Drakes Beach between 9 A.M. and 3 P.M. Tickets are $5 for adults and are free for children 12 and under. No advance reservations are available. The bus leaves approximately every 15 to 20 minutes, according to demand, and runs only in good weather. Call (415) 464-5100 for updates. The last bus leaves Drakes Beach at 3:30 P.M., the lighthouse at 5 P.M., and Chimney Rock at 5:30 P.M.

See the Sir Francis Drake Highway Trailheads section for more information on the lighthouse and Chimney Rock.

Gas Stations
The only gas stations in the area are in the towns of Point Reyes Station and Bolinas, and at the Olema Campground.

VISITOR CENTERS

Bear Valley Visitor Center
Location: Bear Valley Headquarters
Hours: open all year Monday through Friday from 9 A.M. to 5 P.M.; weekends and holidays from 8 A.M. to 5 P.M.; closed December 25
Facilities: Restrooms, water, picnic tables, phone; wheelchair-accessible
Phone: (415) 464-5100

Ken Patrick Visitor Center
Location: Drakes Beach, 30 minutes from Bear Valley off of Sir Francis Drake Highway
Hours: Open weekends and holidays from 10 A.M. to 5 P.M.; closed December 25.
Facilities: Restrooms, water, picnic tables, phone, showers, cafe; wheelchair-accessible
Phone: (415) 669-1250

Lighthouse Visitor Center
Location: Point Reyes headland
Hours: Open Thursday through Monday from 10 A.M. to 4:30 P.M.; closed December 25.
Facilities: Restrooms and water; wheelchair-accessible
Phone: (415) 669-1534

CAMPING AT POINT REYES NATIONAL SEASHORE

Point Reyes National Seashore has four hike-in campgrounds, and several boat-in sites. All require an advance reservation permit.

See the section on Backpacking, pages 197–206, for details on reservations, descriptions of each camp, and suggested backpack trips. All of the camps are also close enough to trailheads to be great dayhike destinations for a picnic or a day at the beach.

See the section on Kayaking, pages 67–69, for details about boat-in camping.

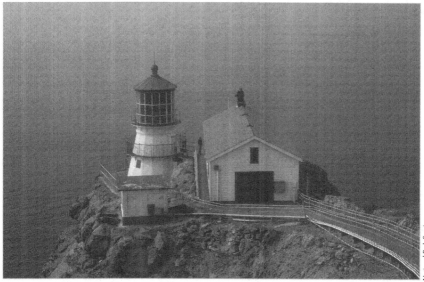

Point Reyes Lighthouse

People often think of fire as a destructive process. We see the damage it can cause to homes and property and the threat it poses to humans and animals. In the natural world, though, fire takes on a vastly different meaning. Until we began to actively suppress fires nearly a century ago, fires regularly occurred in wildlands. Natural fires ignited through lightning and lava flows. Coast Miwok used fire to burn the undergrowth around oak trees, making it easier to gather acorns, and to reduce thick shrub growth, so they could more readily find and dig up bulbs.

Not only an effective tool for managing the land, we now understand that fire is also healthy for the ecosystem. A basic organic process, fire is part of an ecosystem's natural cycle of life and regeneration. Fire complements photosynthesis, in which plants use energy from the sun to convert basic chemical elements—water and carbon dioxide—into new cells. Fire returns this energy back into the atmosphere in the form of smoke, heat, and steam. Additionally, it allows new plants to establish themselves by clearing the land of vegetation and opening the understory to sunlight. Ash from tree litter and other organic debris become fertilizer for seedlings.

However, fire in a populated area can devastate people, communities, and property. The 1995 Vision Fire at Point Reyes was a frightening wake-up call for the National Park and for Marin communities. (See pages 40–42 for more about the Vision Fire.)

Reducing the Risk

The National Park Service and cooperating agencies carry out prescribed burns as a way to reduce hazardous fuels. Burns are a trickier undertaking than thinning and cutting vegetation, since climatic conditions—air quality, wind direction and speed, humidity, and temperature—have to be just right to execute a burn. Many more burns are planned each year than are actually carried out, because of these restrictions.

Point Reyes National Seashore abuts several residential communities. Neighborhoods adjacent to open-space lands and with narrow, tree-lined, winding streets, like those on Inverness Ridge and in Bolinas, run a great risk in the event of a wildfire. The Wildland-Urban Interface Initiative (WUII), a federal fire-management program started in 2001, focuses on cutting back thick vegetation (fuel for fires), educating communities about hazards, and helping neighborhoods with protection. Over 40 community-based projects are underway in Marin alone, funded by the National Park Service and the Bureau of Land Management.

Fire Research

At four sites in and around Point Reyes National Seashore, park researchers are monitoring the effects of prescribed burns on rare plants, nonnative plants, and wildlife. In a study of invasive scotch broom at Drakes Estero, researchers are trying to determine the necessary heat and frequency of fire in order to kill the plant and its hearty seeds (broom seeds can retain their reproductive capacity for up to 30 years!). On Bolinas Ridge, initial studies reveal that fire may encourage the spread of the nonnative velvet grass, a perennial that is rapidly expanding its range and crowding out native species.

Another study on Bolinas Ridge is looking at two rare coastal chaparral species—Mason's ceanothus and Marin manzanita. Like most rare and endangered chaparral species, this ceanothus and manzanita depend on fire for seed germination; they cannot resprout on their own. A study on the health of wildlife after a fire is looking at bobcats, coyotes, mule deer, turkey vultures, and other vertebrates in the Douglas-fir habitat at Firtop on Inverness Ridge.

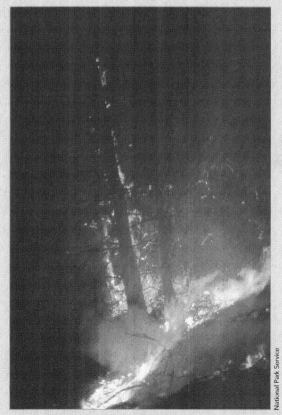

National Park Service

Vision Fire at night

VISITOR REGULATIONS AT POINT REYES NATIONAL SEASHORE

Hikers

- Horses have the right-of-way. Step to the downhill side and greet the rider so the horse knows you are there; do not touch the animals.

Cyclists

- No off-trail riding.
- Do not carry or walk bikes on hiking-only trails.
- Speed limit is 15 miles per hour; slow down on blind curves.
- Bikes yield to hikers and horses.
- Alert other trail users of your approach and indicate how many riders follow.
- Helmets are strongly recommended.

Equestrians

- Horses are allowed on all trails in the park except the Bear Valley, Meadow, and Old Pine trails on weekends and holidays.

Dogs

- Dogs must be on a maximum six-foot leash at all times.
- All hiking trails in the seashore are closed to dogs.
- Limantour, Kehoe, North, and South beaches are open to dogs, except during seasonal closures for habitat protection.
- Dogs are allowed in parking lots and in the Bear Valley Picnic Area.

Fires on the Beach

- Obtain a beach fire permit from the Bear Valley or Drakes Beach visitor center.
- Wood fires are allowed on the sand, away from vegetation. Wood fires are not permitted anywhere else in the park.
- Extinguish fires with water, never by burying coals in the sand.
- Charcoal fires in your own grill are allowed on beaches, and in the grills provided at the Drakes Beach picnic area.

BEAR VALLEY TRAILS AND BEACHES

Park headquarters at Bear Valley is a good first stop on any visit to Point Reyes National Seashore. The main park visitor center is a great resource for information about the park. Several short interpretive walks begin from Bear Valley, and it is the starting point for numerous dayhikes of varying length and for overnights to several of the park campgrounds.

Driving Directions: These directions begin in Olema and Point Reyes Station; to reach these towns, see pages 55–56.

From the junction of Sir Francis Drake Highway and Highway 1 in Olema, make an immediate left on Bear Valley Rd. Continue 0.5 mile to the visitor center road; turn left and go 0.2 mile to a large paved parking area.

From Point Reyes Station, follow Highway 1 through town and just after crossing the green bridge, turn right on Sir Francis Drake Blvd. Go 0.7 mile to Bear Valley Rd., turn left, and continue 1.7 miles to the visitor center road. Turn right and go 0.2 mile to a large paved parking area.

Facilities: Visitor center, restrooms, water, phone, picnic tables, grills; all facilities are wheelchair-accessible (a wheelchair is available for borrowing)

BEAR VALLEY VISITOR CENTER

Exhibits at the visitor center introduce you to the plants, animals, and people of Point Reyes. You can check tide tables and the latest weather forecasts, get wildflower and wildlife updates, and find out about nature programs and other scheduled activities. Free maps and information sheets are available, and the bookstore contains an excellent collection of books about the area. Pick up permits for beach fires and for backcountry and boat-in camping (reservations necessary for camping permits). On request you can watch, in the center's auditorium, a 20-minute slide show, a 22-minute orientation movie about the park, and an 11-minute movie about the lighthouse.

Open weekdays 9 A.M. to 5 P.M.; weekends and holidays 8 A.M. to 5 P.M.

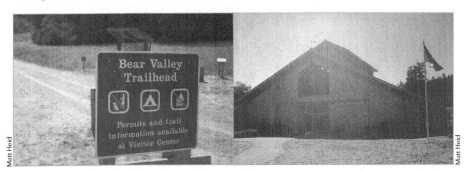

Bear Valley Trailhead   Bear Valley Visitor Center

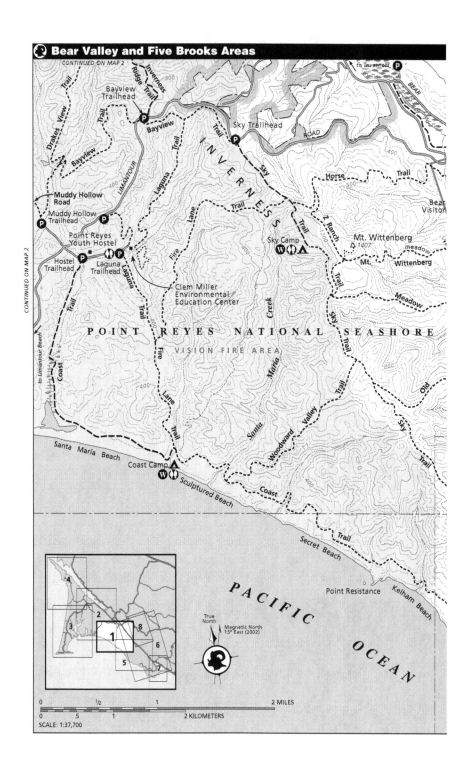

CONTINUED ON MAP 2

to Inverness

Inverness Ridge Trail

Bayview Trailhead

Drakes View Trail

Bayview

Bayview

Muddy Hollow Road

Muddy Hollow Trailhead

Point Reyes Youth Hostel

Hostel Trailhead

Laguna Trailhead

Sky Trailhead

Sky Trail

ROAD

Horse

Trail

Bear Visitor

I N V E R N E S S

LIMANTOUR

Laguna Lane

Laguna Trail

Fire Lane

Laguna

Clem Miller Environmental Education Center

Z Ranch

Sky Camp

Mt. Wittenberg
△ 1407'

meadow

Mt. Wittenberg

Meadow

CONTINUED ON MAP 2

to Limantour Beach

Coast Trail

P O I N T   R E Y E S   N A T I O N A L   S E A S H O R E

VISION FIRE AREA

Fire Lane

Santa Maria Creek

Sky Trail

Old Sky Trail

Santa María Beach

Coast Camp

Sculptured Beach

Woodward Valley

Coast

Secret Beach

Trail

P A C I F I C

Point Resistance

Kelham Beach

O C E A N

True North

Magnetic North 15° East (2002)

0   ½   1   2 MILES
0   .5   1   2 KILOMETERS
SCALE: 1:37,700

Olema

SIR FRANCIS DRAKE

VALLEY

SEE DETAIL

BLVD.

ROAD

Creek

Bear

to Samuel P. Taylor State Park, Fairfax, & San Rafael

Bolinas Ridge Trailhead

Olema

Kule Loklo Valley Center

Bear Valley Trailhead

Trail

Valley

Vedanta Religious Retreat (private)

OLEMA

JAN ANDREAS RIFT ZONE

400

Rift

Zone

Creek

Trail

Pine Trail

Divide Meadow

BEAR

Creek

400

800

VALLEY

RIDGE

Baldy Trail

Bear Valley Trail

Sky Trail

400

Glen Camp Loop

Glen

Coast/ Glen Spur North

Coast

Trail

800

Arch Rock

Millers Point

Wildcat Beach

Coast

Trail

Coast/ Glen Spur South

to Wildcat Camp

Greenpicker Trail

Firtop

Glen Camp

Greenpicker

Stewart Trail

Stewart Trail

Stewart

Trail

Ridge

Old Out Road

Alamea Trail

Stewart Horse Camp

Five Brooks Trailhead

Mill Pond

Five Brooks Ranch Stable

Olema

Olema

Creek

Valley

Trail

Bolema Ridge Trail

Lake Ranch Trail

Mud Lake

GGNRA

400

800

Bear Valley Visitor Center

to Limantour & Inverness

Horse Trail

Kule Loklo

Bear

VALLEY

ROAD

Kule Loklo Trail

Park Headquarters

Morgan Trail

Bear Valley Visitor Center

Morgan Horse Ranch

Red Barn

to Olema

Sky Creek

Woodpecker Trail

Bear Valley Trail

Earthquake Trail

Mt Wittenberg Trail

Rift Zone Trail

0   1/8 MILE
0   0.2 KILOMETER

CONTINUED ON MAP 6

CONTINUED ON MAP 5

CONTINUED ON MAP 5

Bear Valley's W Ranch

Bear Valley is on the site of the former W Ranch, one of the largest historic Point Reyes ranches. Several owners ran the ranch over the years, each according to their own fancy. One owner dammed a creek to create a swimming and boating pond in Bear Valley. Another built a rodeo arena and bleachers in the 1940s and staged three rodeos in what is today the parking lot. W Ranch was the first plot of land the National Park Service acquired after the seashore was established, and the park converted former ranch structures to administration buildings.

INTERPRETIVE TRAILS

Three short educational trails near the visitor center familiarize you with the natural and cultural history of Point Reyes. All are less than 1 mile long, good for first-time visitors to the park, families with small children, tourists with little time to spare, and anyone who wants to learn more about the Coast Miwok, the San Andreas fault, and some of the park's varied natural habitats.

Kule Loklo Trail

Distance: 0.8 mile round trip; trail begins at the northeast edge of the parking lot

Take a short stroll to the replica Coast Miwok village Kule Loklo to find out how the original inhabitants of Point Reyes lived and how their descendants remain connected to Point Reyes today. The village is an important gathering place for local tribe members, who use the replicated roundhouse for ceremonies and celebrate the annual Spring and Big Time festivals every April and July. Hundreds of participants, both tribe members and the general public, join the festivities, watching displays of arrowhead- and basket-making, and tasting

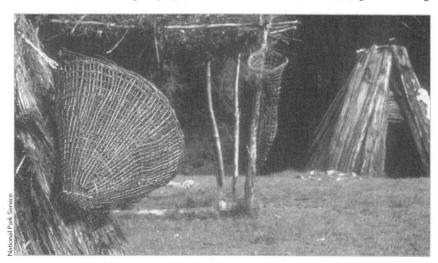

Kule Loklo

traditional foods like frybread and Indian tacos. Kule Loklo, which means Bear Valley in the Coast Miwok language, is both a link to the Coast Miwok past and a contribution to the current and future presence of Native Americans at Point Reyes.

You can take a one-hour ranger-guided tour of Kule Loklo on Sundays at 2 P.M. (meet at the Bear Valley Visitor Center). For information about tours of the roundhouse and California Indian skills classes held at Kule Loklo, contact the Miwok Archeological Preserve of Marin at www.mapom.com or (415) 479-3281. If you are interested in helping maintain Kule Loklo, the park holds a workday on the second Saturday of each month at 10 A.M. For more information, call (415) 464-5131.

An Active Presence

The Federated Indians of Graton Rancheria, which includes Coast Miwok and Southern Pomo groups, became a federally recognized tribe in 2000, and now register some 580 members. To find out more about the Federated Indians of Graton Rancheria and the history of Coast Miwok, visit the tribe's website at www.coastmiwok.com, the Marin Museum of the American Indian site at www.marinindian.com, or contact the Tomales Regional History Center (707) 878-9443.

Earthquake Trail

Distance: 0.6-mile loop; paved, wheelchair-accessible trail begins next to picnic area east of visitor center

Although San Francisco receives the fame for the 1906 earthquake, its epicenter was here in Point Reyes. On this self-guided tour you'll see the fence that was torn apart in the quake as the two sides of the San Andreas fault slid in opposite directions, creating a displacement of about 16 feet in the Olema Valley. The path follows Bear Valley Creek beneath willows and oak trees, and plaques along the route illustrate plate tectonics, tell about the 1906 quake, and give other information about earthquakes. A ranger-guided walk meets at the trailhead every Saturday at 2 P.M.

Woodpecker Trail

Distance: 0.7 mile loop; trail begins at trailhead for Bear Valley Trail

Learn about ecotones (where two plant communities meet), acorn woodpeckers (they can make up to 20,000 holes in one tree!), and the transition from native bunchgrasses to European annuals. Explanatory plaques along this loop trail point out interesting natural features. You climb gently uphill through a stand of trees and then emerge in an open meadow. Views across the meadow take in Black and Barnabe mountains in the distance, and you can see the trough

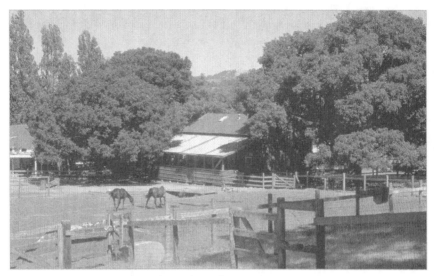
Morgan Horse Ranch at Bear Valley

of the San Andreas fault through Olema Valley. In a rich forest of bay laurel, madrone, live oak, and Douglas-fir trees, you continue climbing along a creekbed, pausing to read about Douglas-firs and winter wrens. Look for hummingbirds feeding on trailing vines of honeysuckle. The trail leaves the forest, skirts a small meadow near the Morgan Horse Ranch, and descends to the trailhead.

Morgan Horse Ranch

A short detour from the Woodpecker Trail takes you to the Morgan Horse Ranch, where you can learn about the history of Morgan horses and watch them in their corral. The first American breed, Morgan horses are known for their speed, endurance, and strength. The Park Service uses these horses in backcountry patrol at Point Reyes and other national parks. Open daily 9 A.M. to 4:30 P.M. (415) 464-5169.

The path next to the corral leads a short distance through a eucalyptus forest to Kule Loklo. You can continue to the Horse Trail, an alternate route to Mt. Wittenberg and Sky Camp.

Bear Valley Trail to
Divide Meadow and Arch Rock

Easy-to-access, fairly level, and exceptionally scenic, this wide trail follows a murmuring creek through a rich forest. Divide Meadow makes a pleasant picnic or rest spot, or even a destination for a short hike. Continue to the coast to visit dramatic Arch Rock. The first part of the Bear Valley Trail is great for bikes, but remember to bring a lock so you can continue to the coast on foot!

Distance: 3.2 miles round trip to Divide Meadow; 8 miles round trip to Arch Rock

Type: Out-and-back

Difficulty: Easy to moderate

Facilities: Bathroom, water, and phone at trailhead; toilet at Divide Meadow, 1.6 miles from trailhead

Regulations: Horses allowed except on weekends and holidays; bikes allowed for the first 3.1 miles to Glen Trail turnoff (bike rack available)

The Bear Valley Trail begins in an open meadow, where you have views east to Bolinas Ridge and beyond to Barnabe Mountain in Samuel P. Taylor Park. Behind you to the north, the rippled slopes of sturdy Black Mountain rise from ranchland. At the far end of the meadow, you pass the trail to Mt. Wittenberg, and your wide, well-graded trail begins to parallel the low ravine of Bear Valley Creek. Under the cover of alders, bay laurels, and elderberry bushes growing along the bank, the temperature drops significantly.

For the next mile and a half, the mostly level trail leads through lush forest. At 0.8 mile you pass the Meadow Trail, which leads 1.7 miles to the ridgetop (see Trip 3). Look for newts crossing the moist trail in the rainy season, and winter wrens darting amid dense tangles of vegetation. Bracken, five-finger, and sword ferns coat the slopes. The heart-shaped leaves of wild ginger (and their flowers, between March and July) grow on the stream bank, and in spring, buttercups, milkmaids, and forget-me-nots sprout along the trail. Just before Divide Meadow at 1.6 miles, the trail climbs slightly to reach the broad, peaceful expanse, ringed by Douglas-fir trees and dappled with oaks.

In the late 19th century, members of elite San Francisco society vacationed at a hunting lodge in Divide Meadow. The wealthy guests (among them was Theodore Roosevelt) hunted bears, mountain lions, and

Fault zones often cause unusual drainage patterns, as is the case along the San Andreas fault in Olema Valley. Bear Valley Creek, which borders the Bear Valley Trail from Divide Meadow to the trailhead, flows north, while Coast Creek, which runs west from Divide Meadow to the ocean, flows south.

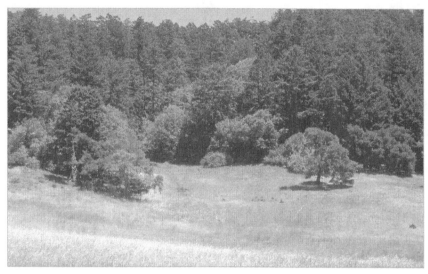
Divide Meadow

deer. Getting to the lodge was an adventure in itself: the men traveled from San Francisco via ferry to Sausalito, by train to Point Reyes Station, and then to Bear Valley by horse and wagon.

To reach the coast, continue on the Bear Valley Trail as it gently descends and then levels along alder-lined Coast Creek, which flows to the ocean. After 1.5 miles beyond Divide Meadow (3.1 from the trailhead), you meet a junction with the Glen Trail, where bicyclists must leave their bikes and proceed to the coast on foot (bike racks available). The Glen Trail climbs south out of Bear Valley to reach Glen Camp and connect with trails in the Five Brooks area (see Trip 6).

Hidden Gardens of Mosses and Lichens

The Bear Valley Trail is an ideal place to discover the hidden world of mosses and lichens—organisms that often go unnoticed by humans, but are full of marvel and worth a few extra minutes on the trail. One easy-to-notice inhabitant is the lacy green lichen that hangs from the branches of Douglas-fir and bishop pine, commonly called "witches hair" or "old man's beard" (but often misidentified as "Spanish moss").

Classified as part of the fungal kingdom, lichens are not plants, but rather a unique partnership between a fungus and a green alga or a blue-green bacterium. The partnership is often called a mutualistic relationship, because both partners benefit. The fungal partner, the main body of the lichen, protects the algal mate and absorbs water and minerals, while the alga provides the organism with food through photosynthesis.

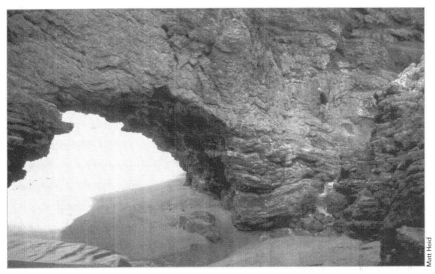

Arch Rock

In deep shade and alongside lush riparian vegetation, the Bear Valley Trail continues its westward course for 0.9 mile to reach the coast. You soon sense the proximity of the ocean, as the trail becomes increasingly sandy. After a gentle rise, you emerge on a low, open bluff at the mouth of the valley. About 50 feet above the sea, you are on a marine terrace that extends from Bolinas Mesa to Limantour, although a large landslide obscures the terrace for several miles south of Bear Valley.

The Bear Valley Trail ends at a T-junction with the Coast Trail. Veer left and follow the Coast Trail south for a few hundred yards to a small, right-branching spur to Arch Rock. The narrow trail leads 0.1 mile to a spectacular promontory above the sea, where you can look down on the rocky beach below. On a clear day, you'll have views from Chimney Rock to Double Point and out to the Farallon Islands.

A small and precarious trail (not an official park trail) leads down the inland side of the promontory and follows Coast Creek a few hundred feet to the beach. From here, you can see the tunnel, or arch, where the stream meets the ocean. At low tide, you may be able to cross the creek and explore the small beach. **Warning:** Proceed with great caution. The trail to the creek is steep and eroding and the crossing can be slippery. Watch the tide to avoid becoming trapped on the beach.

When you return to the junction with the Coast Trail, you can continue south for about a quarter of a mile to Millers Point, a great place for a picnic. Named for congressman Clem Miller, who played a pivotal role in establishing Point

Arch Rock is a classic sea arch, formed by years of wave and water erosion. Continued erosion will eventually wear away the natural bridge between the rock and the headland, isolating the rock entirely and creating a sea stack.

Reyes as a national seashore, this grassy bluff affords a different perspective on Arch Rock and more great views.

You can return to the trailhead via the Bear Valley Trail for a round trip of 8.2 miles, or, if after this leisurely walk through Bear Valley and a rest at Arch Rock, you're up for a more rigorous return route, you can take the Coast Trail north to the Sky or Woodward Valley trails. Both trails climb Inverness Ridge and present descent options on the Meadow or Mt. Wittenberg trails. These routes make for round trips of 11 and 12.8 miles. (See Trips 3 and 4.)

Trip 2 Bear Valley to Mt. Wittenberg

You'll get a taste of inland and coastal environments on this short but steep trip to the highest point in the seashore, first in the mixed forest on the eastern flank of Mt. Wittenberg and then on the open seaside slopes. A picnic or rest stop on the 1407-foot summit affords exhilarating views of the coastline.

Distance: 4.4 miles round trip
Type: Out-and-back (with loop options)
Difficulty: Moderate
Facilities: Bathroom, water, and phone at trailhead
Regulations: Horses allowed except on weekends and holidays on the Bear Valley, Meadow, and Old Pine trails; no bikes; no dogs

Begin on the Bear Valley Trail in the open meadow at the far end of the parking lot. Take in views east of Bolinas Ridge and beyond to Barnabe Mountain in Samuel P. Taylor Park, and north of Black Mountain. Turn right on the Mt. Wittenberg Trail (sometimes called the Sky Trail, depending on the map or trail sign), 0.2 mile from the trailhead.

You immediately begin to ascend through a forest of Douglas-firs, bay laurel, and tanbark oak. Leafy branches of hazelnut and huckleberry bushes drape above immense fronds of sword fern. The trail crosses a large clearing, which is gradually becoming a forest of small Douglas-fir trees. After a brief respite from the climb, you ascend again through tree cover to reach the open hillside just below Mt. Wittenberg. You'll have your first views of the coastline as you crest the rise, where the grassy slope teems with wildflowers in spring.

At a junction here, turn right on a small path that leads 0.2 mile to the summit. A 360-degree view of Point Reyes and the surrounding area takes in the coastline, Drakes and Limantour esteros, Tomales Bay, Black Mountain, Olema Valley and Bolinas Ridge; on especially clear days, you might see Mts. St. Helena, Diablo, and Tamalpais.

When you have enjoyed the view and regained your energy, retrace your steps to the junction to find several options for returning to the trailhead or extending your hike. Backpackers will want to head down the slope on the Sky Trail and continue to Sky Camp; those who have arranged a shuttle trip to the Sky Trailhead will also want to take this route. To return to Bear Valley on a different route, turn right on the Z Ranch Trail, and then right again when it meets the Horse Trail (not just for horses), which you follow back to the visitor center.

Bear Valley to Meadow to Old Pine, Baldy, or the Coast

Climb shaded paths through a lush forest from Bear Valley to reach Inverness Ridge, travel the ridgeline beneath towering Douglas-firs with views of the coastline, and return along the creekside Bear Valley Trail. To turn this exceptional hike into a full-day excursion through varied terrain and vegetation, you can continue on the Sky Trail along the ridge, take in fantastic views as you descend to the coast, visit Arch Rock, and then stroll back to the trailhead on the Bear Valley Trail. After you climb the ridge, the route is level or descending for the rest of the hike.

Distance: 6.8 miles via Old Pine; 8.9 miles via Baldy; 11 miles to the coast and back
Type: Semi-loop
Difficulty: Moderate to strenuous
Facilities: Bathroom, water, and phone at Bear Valley Trailhead; toilets at Divide Meadow
Regulations: Horses allowed except on weekends and holidays on the Bear Valley, Meadow, and Old Pine trails; no bikes; no dogs

Across the meadow at the trailhead, you have views of Bolinas Ridge and Barnabe Mountain; behind you, Black Mountain rises in the distance. At the far end of the meadow, you pass the trail to Mt. Wittenberg and soon begin to parallel Bear Valley Creek. Your wide, well-graded route enters the cover of alders, bay laurels, and elderberry bushes that grow on the stream banks; oaks and Douglas-firs grow on higher slopes.

At 0.8 mile, turn right on the Meadow Trail and cross the wooden bridge over the creek. The trail climbs steeply through a rich forest of Douglas-fir, tanbark oak, delicate hazelnut, and musky California bay laurel, with chain fern, evergreen huckleberry, thimbleberry, and gooseberry beneath. You soon reach an open meadow lined with Douglas-fir, and as the grade lessens you have views to the east of Bolinas Ridge and distant Mt. Tamalpais.

Because of the cool, riparian habitat along the creek, the Bear Valley Trail is a great place to identify ferns that are common in Point Reyes. In winter, look for California polypody and licorice fern (*polypodium californicum* and *p. plycyrrhiza*) growing on tree trunks and downed logs. You won't even notice these small, shade-loving ferns after they die back in summer, waiting to reappear again next winter.

At the ridgetop junction (2.3 miles from the trailhead), you turn left on the Sky Trail. (You could go right on the Sky Trail to Sky Camp or to ascend Mt. Wittenberg from here.) Light-green lichen dangles from Douglas-fir branches, high above the rich understory of western sword fern, Douglas iris, and red elderberry. Heading toward the ocean along the crest of Inverness Ridge, you catch glimpses of the spectacular coastline through the trees.

At 3.1 miles from the trailhead, you pass a small clearing where the Woodward Valley Trail branches left and heads for the coast. A few short ascents and descents beyond, you reach a junction with the Old Pine Trail, where you turn left and continue through the Douglas-fir forest. Soon, huckleberry and elderberry bushes and honeysuckle vines outnumber the fir trees. On a gentle descent, you cross a small meadow surrounded by high trees and, after 1.9 miles, arrive at Divide Meadow. Turn left on the smooth Bear Valley Trail, which offers a nearly level return to the trailhead along Bear Valley Creek.

To extend this route, continue south on the gently undulating Sky Trail past the junction with the Old Pine Trail. As you near the coast, you notice subtle changes in the vegetation and soil. Coyote bush, sticky monkeyflower, blackberry, wild cucumber, and poison oak become prominent as you reach the Baldy

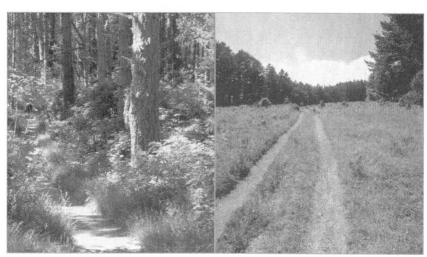

Old Pine Trail   Meadow Trail

Trail junction, 1.4 miles beyond the Old Pine Trail, and views of the coast peek through the vegetation with increasing frequency. Turn left on the Baldy Trail to meet the Bear Valley Trail and return to the trailhead in 4.3 miles.

For a full-day coastal hike, stay on the Sky Trail and begin the long descent to the coast, with expansive views every step of the way. Turn left on the Coast Trail, and follow it half a mile to Arch Rock and the junction with the Bear Valley Trail, your return route. You soon enter the shade of alder trees along the lush bed of Coast Creek. The Glen Trail branches right after 0.9 mile from the coast, a possible route to Five Brooks. At 1.5 miles beyond, your trail ascends gently to Divide Meadow, where oaks provide a bit of shade on the broad expanse. The meadow is a perfect spot for a rest, but you are only 1.6 miles from the trailhead, which you will reach after a brief descent and a level, shaded course along Bear Valley Creek.

Bear Valley to the Coast via Mt. Wittenberg and the Woodward Valley trails

Trip 4

This long hike visits the best of the Bear Valley area. Skirt the seashore's highest point and then descend to the ocean with great views of the coastline. On the level trail along the coastal bluff look for wildflowers, whales, and sea lions. Before heading inland along a creek, you can visit the dramatic rocky promontory of Arch Rock.

Distance: 12.8 miles
Type: Loop
Difficulty: Strenuous
Facilities: Bathroom, water, and phone at trailhead; toilet at Divide Meadow
Regulations: Horses allowed except on weekends and holidays on the Bear Valley Trail; no bikes; no dogs

Begin on the Bear Valley Trail at the far end of the parking lot. Take in views east of Bolinas Ridge and beyond to Barnabe Mountain in Samuel P. Taylor Park; behind you is majestic Black Mountain. Skirt the broad meadow for 0.2 mile and then turn right on the Mt. Wittenberg Trail (sometimes called the Sky Trail, depending on the map or trail sign).

A forest of Douglas-firs, bay laurel, and tanbark oak shade the trail as it begins a steep climb up the mountainside. In the understory, hazelnut and huckleberry bushes drape over large fronds of sword fern. The trail crosses a large clearing, encroached upon by small Douglas-firs, and the grade briefly eases. You are soon climbing again through tree cover, but shortly emerge on the open hillside just below Mt. Wittenberg. From the junction on this grassy, wildflower-covered slope, you'll have your first views of the coastline.

Follow the Sky Trail downslope from the junction, taking in views of Drakes Bay. At the next junction, 0.4 mile beyond, continue straight (west) on the Sky Trail. (The Meadow Trail veers left here and returns to the Bear Valley Trail, and the Sky Trail to Sky Camp makes a sharp right turn and heads east.)

As you head toward the ocean along the crest of Inverness Ridge, Douglas-firs tower above and light-green lichen, nurtured by thick summer fogs and rainy winters, hangs from their branches. Western sword fern, red elderberry, and evergreen huckleberry adorn the trailside. You descend to a small clearing, surrounded by high trees, and strike out for the coast on the Woodward Valley Trail. Across the meadow, the trail enters a dense alley of small Douglas-fir trees and soon begins its mostly descending route. On a delightful and varied course, you pass through shaded forest and open coastal-scrub vegetation of sticky monkeyflower, coyote bush, ceanothus, blackberry, and wild cucumber. Charred tree trunks remain standing among vigorous new growth.

Fog can create up to 10 inches of precipitation a year on Inverness Ridge. In summer, moisture dripping from tree cover and tall grasses often makes the trail as muddy as after a winter rain.

From the Woodward Valley Trail, you have a good view of the burned tree trunks that dot the coastal slopes, evidence of the 1995 Vision Fire. The fire enveloped 12,354 acres surrounding Mt. Vision, burning 45 homes and 15 percent of Point Reyes National Seashore. Although the burnt trees are the only obvious remnant, the vibrant growth that surrounds them also resulted from the fire.

Your first view of the ocean, appearing suddenly beyond the folds of the coastal slopes, may take your breath away. Even more spectacular views emerge after a brief climb to a small knoll, where you'll see south to Double Point and north to Chimney Rock. The trail wraps around to the western side of the knoll, and begins to descend an eroded path. You soon turn left on the Coast Trail (5.2 miles from the trailhead), a former ranch road that travels the ancient marine terrace a couple of hundred feet above the ocean. On this level, step-like stretch of land, you follow the Coast Trail south for 3 miles. Coyote bush, blackberry, wild cucumber, tall bushes of ceanothus, and low-growing grasses flank the trail, and in spring, the blue blossoms of Douglas iris put on an elegant show, accompanied by small yellow sun cups and pink checkerbloom.

A spur path to Sculptured Beach shortly branches right, marked by a small sign almost hidden among ceanothus bushes (see side trip). After 2 miles or so, you pass the shale promontory of Point Resistance, where offshore rocks attract pelagic birds like common murres. Continuing on, you reach a large eucalyptus,

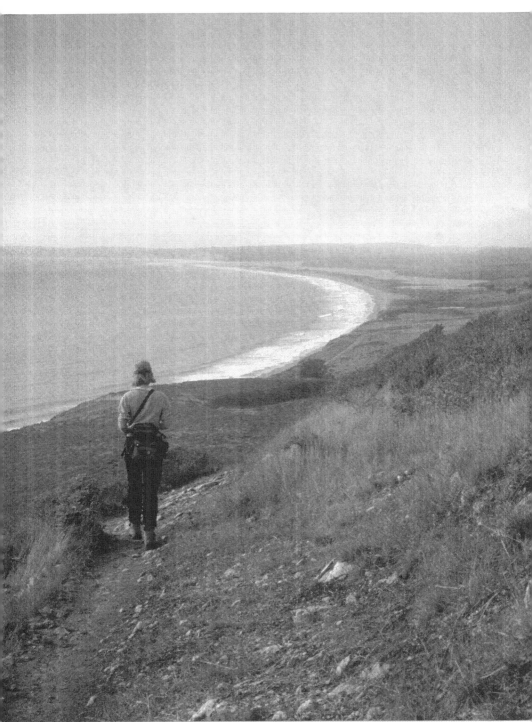

View of Limantour Beach and Drakes Bay from the Woodward Valley Trail

the last remnant of Y Ranch, and an access trail to Kelham Beach (see side trip). Cross a bridge over a small creek that drains from the ridge to the ocean. About half a mile beyond, you pass the Sky Trail and, in another half a mile, reach the Bear Valley Trail near Arch Rock (8.6 miles from the trailhead).

Side Trips to Sculptured and Kelham Beaches

Eroding ochre cliffs enclose Sculptured Beach, forming dramatically contoured canyons behind the sand. Tidepools thrive in the layered rocks near the water. When the tide is very low (minus), you can go south along the beach to visit Secret Beach, but you'll have to return to Sculptured Beach to continue your route on the Coast Trail, since Secret Beach's steep cliffs are unscalable. Be aware of the tide because you can easily become trapped on Secret Beach.

Farther south along the Coast Trail, you can make another short side trip to reach mile-long Kelham Beach. At low tide you can usually walk on the beach south to Arch Rock and north to Point Resistance.

Return on the Bear Valley Trail, following the lush bed of Coast Creek in the shade of alder. You pass the Glen Trail after 0.9 mile from the coast, and nearly 1.5 miles beyond you ascend the gentle downslope of Divide Meadow, where oaks provide a bit of shade on the broad expanse. You are only 1.6 miles from the trailhead, which you will reach after a brief descent and a level, shaded course along Bear Valley Creek.

Bear Valley to the Coast via the Glen Trail

This variation on the Bear Valley Trail to Arch Rock provides outstanding views from the coastal bluff, a good whale-watching vantage point, and a hillside full of spring wildflowers.

Distance: 9.9 miles
Type: Semi-loop
Difficulty: Moderate
Facilities: Bathroom, water, phone at trailhead; toilets at Divide Meadow
Regulations: Horses allowed except on weekends and holidays; bikes allowed for the first 3.1 miles to Glen Trail turnoff (bike rack available)

The Bear Valley Trail begins in an open meadow, where you have views east to Bolinas Ridge and beyond to the peak of Barnabe Mountain in Samuel P. Taylor Park. Behind you, to the north, sturdy Black Mountain rises from ranchland. At the far end of the meadow, you pass the trail to Mt. Wittenberg and continue on your wide, well-graded route along the low ravine of Bear Valley Creek. Alders, bay laurels, and elderberry bushes on the creek bank and oaks and Douglas-firs on higher slopes keep the trail cool.

For the next mile and a half, a lush forest encloses the mostly level trail. At 0.8 mile you pass the Meadow Trail, which leads 1.7 miles to the ridgetop (see Trip 3). The trail comes alive in the rainy season, with newts crossing the moist trail, winter wrens darting amid dense tangles of vegetation, and bracken, five-finger, and sword ferns coating the slopes. The heart-shaped leaves of wild ginger (and their flowers, between March and July) grow on the stream banks, and in spring, buttercups, milkmaids, and forget-me-nots border the trail.

The trail climbs slightly to reach Divide Meadow at 1.6 miles, a broad, peaceful expanse, ringed by Douglas-fir trees and dappled with oaks. The Old Pine Trail branches right to climb Inverness Ridge. Stay on the Bear Valley Trail as it gently descends from the meadow and then levels to continue along alder-lined Coast Creek, which flows into the ocean. After 3.1 miles from the trailhead, you reach the Glen Trail. If you're on a bike, you can lock your bike here at the rack to proceed on foot for the rest of this trip.

The wide, shaded Glen Trail immediately crosses Coast Creek and begins to climb out of Bear Valley, leaving the lush riparian vegetation of alder, elderberry, and ferns. You cross a level meadow and then climb again through a drier forest to meet the Glen Camp Loop Trail, which goes left toward the camp. You continue under Douglas-fir, bay laurel, and hazelnut, and soon branch right on the Coast/Glen Spur to meet the Coast Trail in a grassy meadow.

Head west (right) on the Coast Trail, alongside low shrubs of coyote bush and a tangle of blackberry and poison oak. The trail begins to descend gradually and emerges from the bushes. On a coastal hillside swathed with spring wildflowers in bright yellows, blues, and oranges, you have fabulous views of the ocean, Drakes Bay, and Chimney Rock. You reach a small knoll just to the left of the trail, a good rest and view spot, and then descend more steeply. Eroded in patches, the trail soon reaches Millers Point at the coast and curves to the right to heads north along the bluff.

As you approach the mouth of Coast Creek, lush vegetation lines the trail, interspersed with the rounded white umbels of cow parsnip and the white flowers or red fruits of elderberry. Beyond a wooden bridge over the creek, the trail rises to a junction with a spur path to Arch Rock. Turn left for a 0.1-mile side trip to the dramatic promontory, or go right to meet the Bear Valley Trail (0.1 mile in the other direction). At the junction with the Bear Valley Trail, you will have come 5.8 miles from the trailhead and can make an easy return along this wide, multi-use trail.

Under the shade of alder and bay laurel trees, the trail follows the lush bed of Coast Creek. You pass the Glen Trail after 0.9 mile from the coast, and then retrace your steps to the trailhead, passing Divide Meadow along the way.

Rift Zone Trail

The San Andreas rift zone (a collection of faults that includes the major San Andreas fault) is the meeting point of the Pacific Plate, on which Point Reyes peninsula lies, and the mainland North American Plate. This easy trail follows the fault's route through Olema Valley, across fields and through forests that vibrate with green in winter and spring—from the grasses in the pastures, to the lichens hanging from bare tree branches, and the delicate new leaves on bushes and trees. During the wet season, the pastures are often muddy, and you may have to dodge cow dung. After a long, dry summer the trail can be very dusty.

Distance: 4.5 miles one-way to Five Brooks
Type: Out-and-back or shuttle
Difficulty: Easy
Facilities: Bathroom, water, and phone at Bear Valley Trailhead; toilet and water at Five Brooks Trailhead
Regulations: No dogs. The trail crosses land that belongs to the Vedanta Society; observe their rules: open 8 A.M. to 2 hours before sunset; no bikes, no fires or smoking, no camping or picnicking, no hunting, close livestock gates.

The Rift Zone Trail starts out across the broad meadow at the Bear Valley Trailhead, signed FIVE BROOKS. On your left you can see the informative plaques along the Earthquake Trail (a good trail to take before this one for some background on the San Andreas fault). You soon enter the shade of bay laurel and oak trees and dip into the bed of Bear Valley Creek.

Live oaks are scarce on the Point Reyes peninsula, but those that do grow here, usually in protected inland areas of the peninsula, draw migrating land-birds in spring. The convergence of the bay and oak forest and the riparian woodland along this section of the Rift Zone Trail provides habitat for several bird species not frequently seen on the peninsula. Look for Nuttall's woodpecker, plain titmouse, lazuli bunting, and house wren.

Cross a wooden bridge over the creek and ascend a small knoll, crowned by beautifully shaped live oaks. On the other side of the rise, you go through a livestock gate and cross a meadow where deer often gather. Ahead, a row of eucalyptus and Monterey cypress line the road to the Vedanta Society Retreat.

Two gates, on either side of the road, mark the entrance to their land, which you will be on for the next 3 miles. (Please stay on the trail.)

Just beyond the gates, cattle graze in a large field where the grassy trail is hard to discern at times, but occasional posts mark the way. Go through a gate on the far side of the field and turn left on an old farm road. The next 2 miles of trail follow this wide dirt road through varied countryside. In cool forests, bay laurel, Douglas-fir, live oak, and alder trees shade an understory of moist ferns and huckleberry. The trail skirts tule- and reed-lined marshes and crosses peaceful meadows. Although they may be hard to spot amongst the tree cover, listen for the calls of landbirds that flock to these forests on their migratory journeys.

Soon after passing a sign marking the other boundary of the Vedanta Society property, you switchback down a short hill and cross a creek on a wooden bridge. Follow signs to continue on the Rift Zone Trail. Beyond another meadow and a creek ford (be prepared for some mud in wet weather), you reach Stewart Horse Camp in a broad clearing. Stay on the Rift Zone Trail, returning temporarily to forest cover and passing a run-down cottage adorned with shells. Shortly, the trail meets the wide path that circles the mill pond at Five Brooks. Turn left to reach the parking lot.

The Vedanta religion is based on the final books of the Vedas (Indo-Aryan scriptures), called the Upanishads. The teachings of Vedanta emphasize the Spirit as the essence of all living things. The society, with headquarters in San Francisco, established a small monastic community in Olema in 1946, which has functioned as a retreat center since the 1970s. The center occupies over 2000 acres, previously owned by James McMillan Shafter. Shafter's stately mansion, built in 1869, is now the center's headquarters.

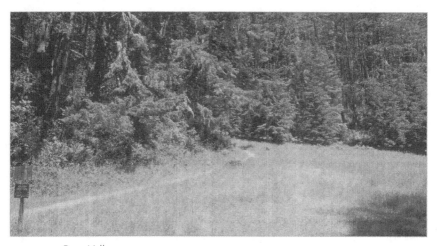

Bear Valley

LIMANTOUR ROAD TRAILS AND BEACHES

Driving to a trailhead on Limantour Road can be a trip in itself. The road climbs Inverness Ridge, and then descends west to Limantour Beach, offering spectacular views across the undulating coastal slopes and Drakes Bay to Chimney Rock at the tip of Point Reyes. Trailheads along the road offer starting points for hikes along the ridge, to Bear Valley, and to the coast. With just a short walk from the Sky Trailhead, you can spend a night at the ridgetop Sky Camp.

Limantour Road recalls the early days of Point Reyes National Seashore, when planners envisioned roads throughout the park that would serve an auto-oriented seashore recreation area. Limantour Road was the only major construction project

SWINDLES, SCHEMES, AND SUBDIVISIONS IN LIMANTOUR'S PAST

The Limantour area was named for a French trader and Mexican citizen who sailed his trading ship up the California coast in 1841. He had intended to stop in San Francisco, but missed the Golden Gate and ran aground on the sand spit today called Limantour Spit. Leaving his cargo of French silk brocades, clothing, perfumes, brandies, and sweetmeats on the beach, Limantour made his way by land to San Francisco. After returning to collect his goods, Limantour remained in the area and proceeded to swindle land buyers out of hundreds of thousands of dollars by forging land grants. He escaped to Mexico with his fortune before the federal government caught up with him.

By the 1850s the Shafter brothers owned most of the Point Reyes peninsula. In 1889, James McMillan Shafter was struggling to recover his debt from investments in the North Coast Pacific Railroad. To pay off his creditors, he turned to his only remaining asset—land. Shafter proposed a sprawling suburban paradise and put up for sale 13,300 subdivided acres on Drake's Bay.

Although Shafter's scheme for the Limantour area was a flop, less than 100 years later developers once again set their sights on Limantour. In 1960, Marin County supervisors approved plans for a subdivision on Limantour Spit— Drakes Beach Estates. A San Francisco newspaper reported in 1961 that the "stakes are up, with fluttering blue and red ribbons attached, on the half-acre homesites. Architects and engineers are at work on plans to dredge a small boat harbor, lay out a golf course, and erect a Carmel-type commercial development." Developers began to level hills and to construct roads, sewer lines, and homes. They had already built 18 homes in the subdivision when the National Park Service was finally able to purchase the property in 1963. Park personnel now occupy the few houses that remain on the bluff above the beach.

in the original park plans that was implemented, although its location on steep and unstable terrain very near to the San Andreas fault provoked many objections.

In 1995, the Vision Fire swept across the Limantour area. In the months after the fire, it was a desolate and scarred landscape of burned bishop pines and shrubs. After plentiful rain the following spring, the hills were already green and sprouting new vegetation. Many years later, the effects of the Vision Fire on the Limantour ecosystem are still apparent, although vigorous growth abounds, and spring wildflowers and healthy wildlife populations thrive here. Plant succession and regrowth is fascinating to observe as you hike these trails. For more information on the Vision Fire, see pages 40–42.

Original plans for the national seashore also called for extensive development of the Limantour–Drakes Estero area—roads, parking lots, food concession-aires, bath houses, campgrounds with over 500 sites, fishing piers, and charter boat rentals. A providential shift in values from recreation to preservation averted a theme-park atmosphere at Limantour, and in the rest of the national seashore. Today, an expanse of undeveloped open space, hiking trails and animal pathways crisscrosses the coastal scrublands from Inverness Ridge to Limantour Beach. The Limantour area lies within the Phillip Burton Wilderness Area.

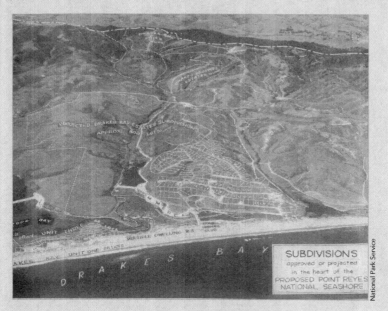

Drakes Bay development subdivisions map

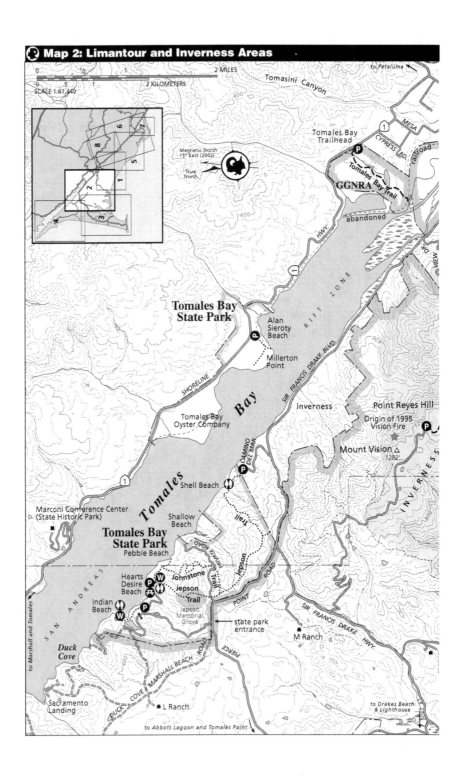

SCALE 1:61,440

0   .5   1   2 MILES
0   .5   1   2 KILOMETERS

to Petaluma

Tomasini Canyon

Magnetic North
15° East (2002)

True North

Tomales Bay Trailhead

GGNRA

Tomales Bay Trail

abandoned

MESA

CYPRESS RD.

railroad

VIEW DR.

HWY. 1

RIFT ZONE

Tomales Bay State Park

Alan Sieroty Beach

Millerton Point

SIR FRANCIS DRAKE BLVD.

SHORELINE

Tomales Bay

Tomales Bay Oyster Company

Inverness

Point Reyes Hill

Origin of 1995 Vision Fire

Mount Vision △ 1282'

INVERNESS

CAMINO DEL MAR

Shell Beach

Tomales Bay Trail

Marconi Conference Center (State Historic Park)

Shallow Beach

HWY. 1

Tomales Bay State Park
Pebble Beach

Johnstone Trail

Jepson Trail

POINT

SIR FRANCIS DRAKE HWY.

Hearts Desire Beach

Jepson Trail

Jepson Memorial Grove

state park entrance

M Ranch

Indian Beach

SAN ANDREAS

Duck Cove

to Marshall and Tomales

DUCK COVE / MARSHALL BEACH ROAD

PIERCE

Sacramento Landing

L Ranch

to Drakes Beach & Lighthouse

to Abbots Lagoon and Tomales Point

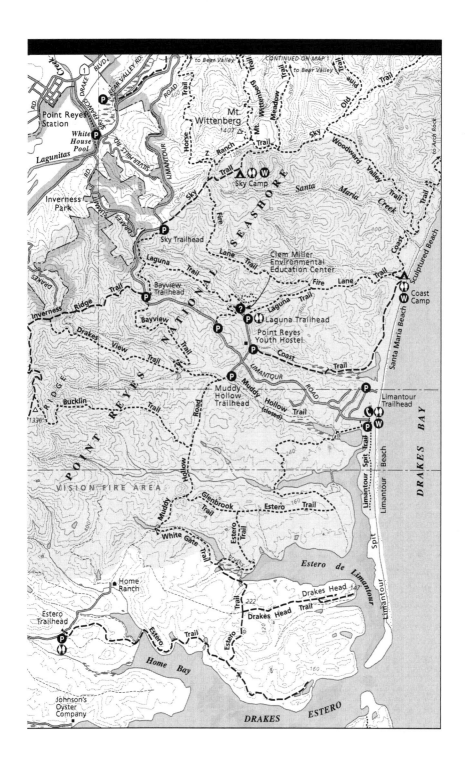

On the crest of Inverness Ridge, the Sky Trailhead provides an easier starting point for hikes to Mt. Wittenberg and along the ridge than the Bear Valley Trailhead, because you gain most of the elevation on the drive. It is also a good starting point for loop hikes to the coast.

Driving Directions: From the Bear Valley Visitor Center, return to Bear Valley Road. Turn left and drive 1.5 miles to the Limantour Road. Turn left again and follow the road for 3.5 miles to the Sky Trailhead on the west side of Limantour Road.
Facilities: None

Mt. Wittenberg via the Horse and Z Ranch trails

Trip 7

This modest climb to the seashore's highest point offers the same spectacular views from the top, explores the less-traveled Horse and Z Ranch trails, and visits Sky Camp on the return.

Distance: 2.1 miles to Mt. Wittenberg; 4.6 total, returning on the Sky Trail
Type: Loop
Difficulty: Moderate
Facilities: Toilet, water, picnic tables, and hitch rail at Sky Camp
Regulations: No bikes or dogs; horses allowed

Begin on the wide Sky Trail as it climbs south from the parking lot. On a steady grade along this old ranch road you pass through open scrub vegetation into a shady Douglas-fir forest with a lush understory. After 0.7 mile, the Fire Lane Trail branches right, and just beyond, you turn left on the Horse Trail.

Contrary to its name, the Horse Trail is not just for horses and is actually quite pleasant for hikers, especially this short section that leads to the eastern side of Mt. Wittenberg. After a brief, gentle climb, the narrow trail levels and edges a steep canyon. Through the dense vegetation, you have views northeast across Tomales Bay to the peaks beyond.

In just 0.4 mile, you reach a junction with the Z Ranch Trail. The Horse Trail goes left to continue for 1.7 miles to Bear Valley, and you turn right on the Z Ranch Trail, headed for Mt. Wittenberg. The wide, level trail skirts the forested slopes of the mountain and passes above the Sky Trail and Sky Camp. On clear days, you'll have spectacular views of Drakes Bay beyond charred tree trunks, remnants of the Vision Fire that burned these slopes in 1995.

After 0.7 mile on the Z Ranch Trail, you arrive at a junction in an open meadow on the peak's flank. The Mt. Wittenberg Trail from Bear Valley converges with a connector to the Sky Trail and a short path to the peak. Turn left and ascend the narrow 0.2-mile path to the broad summit plateau, a great place for a picnic lunch, a nap, or just an extended rest. Take in the 360-degree view of the Point Reyes peninsula, including Limantour and Drakes esteros, and of Tomales Bay, Black Mountain, Olema Valley, and Bolinas Ridge. If the weather is clear, you'll see to Mt. St. Helena, Mt. Diablo, and Mt. Tamalpais.

Z Ranch, the highest elevation ranch on the peninsula, occupied the site of present-day Sky Camp. All that remains of the ranch, whose first tenants were the Wittenbergs, is an old spring and some cypress and eucalyptus trees that mark the location of the buildings.

After you've had your fill of views, retrace your steps to the last junction and follow signs to the Sky Trail, 0.4 mile down the mountain. Turn right on the Sky Trail and follow the wide ranch road on a mostly level route through the forest, with open, viewful patches. In just over half a mile, you reach campsites on open slopes at Sky Camp, where you'll find a toilet, picnic tables, and hitch rail. (For information about camping, see pages 197–206.) Beyond the camp, the trail continues through a landscape of burned tree trunks amid lush vegetation, evidence of the Mt. Vision Fire. You pass the Horse Trail after 0.5 mile from the camp and retrace your steps to the trailhead.

Trip 8 | Woodward Valley Trail to the Coast; return on the Fire Lane Trail

This loop trip reaches the coast on the Woodward Valley Trail—one of the most delightful trails in the seashore—and visits Sculptured Beach on a short detour. Also a good backpacking trip, this route passes both Sky and Coast camps.

Distance: 8.6 miles
Type: Loop
Difficulty: Moderate to strenuous
Facilities: Toilet, water, picnic tables, and hitch rail at Sky and Coast camps
Regulations: No bikes or dogs; horses allowed

Begin on the Sky Trail, a wide old ranch road that heads south from the parking area. A steady climb leads through open scrub vegetation into a shady Douglas-fir forest with a lush understory. The trail levels after 0.7 mile, and you pass the Fire Lane Trail. Shortly thereafter, the Horse Trail branches left, and

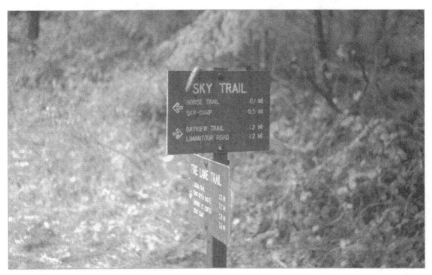

Sky and Fire Lane trails junction

your trail descends slightly, with views of the coast to the west. The Vision Fire cleared these slopes in 1995, leaving only burned tree trunks. The vibrant vegetation that surrounds these trees today was reinvigorated by the burn.

Just 1.3 miles from the trailhead, you reach Sky Camp, with campsites, toilets, picnic tables, and a hitch rail. (For information about camping, see pages 197–206.) The Sky Trail continues beyond the camp, along the western flank of Mt. Wittenberg. After 0.6 mile from the camp, you reach a junction with the Meadow Trail, and a connector trail that leads to the Mt. Wittenberg Trail and to the peak.

Continue on the Sky Trail, heading toward the ocean along the crest of Inverness Ridge. Douglas-firs tower above you, and a rich understory of Douglas iris, western sword fern, red elderberry, and evergreen huckleberry adorns the trailside. Light-green moss drips from the fir branches, nurtured by thick summer fog and rainy winters. Through the trees, you catch glimpses of the spectacular coastline.

The Sky Trail dips into a glade surrounded by high trees, where you branch right on the Woodward Valley Trail (2.7 miles from the trailhead). Cross the meadow to enter a dense alley of small Douglas-fir trees. The trail soon begins its mostly descending route to the coast, delightful and varied, alternately passing through shaded forest and open coastal-scrub vegetation of sticky monkeyflower, coyote bush, ceanothus, blackberry, and morning glory. Charred tree trunks stand among vigorous new growth.

Your first view of the ocean, beyond the folds of the coastal slopes, appears suddenly as you emerge from tree cover. After a brief climb to a small knoll, you'll have even more spectacular views—south to Double Point and north to Chimney Rock.

The Woodward Valley Trail wraps around the knoll and continues a steady descent, winding down the open coastal slope to reach the Coast Trail, 4.7 miles from the trailhead.

Side Trip to Sculptured Beach
A brief jaunt (1.1 miles round trip) south (left) along the Coast Trail brings you to a short path marked by a small sign among ceanothus bushes. The path descends to Sculptured Beach, where eroding ochre cliffs form contoured canyons behind the sand. Complexly layered rocks provide habitat for tidepool life. At low tide, you can go north on the beach to Coast Camp, and rejoin the described hike there. At *really* low tide (minus), you can go south along the beach to visit Secret Beach.

Turn right on the Coast Trail and head north, taking in dramatic views of Drakes Bay, Limantour Beach, and Chimney Rock. The trail heads inland along the gully of Santa Maria Creek, where riparian willows and alders line the creek and overhang the trail. You cross the watercourse on a wooden bridge, and climb gradually past abundant ceanothus bushes, deliciously fragrant in spring. A craggy granite outcropping protrudes from the hillside above. The trail soon drops into Coast Camp, with a toilet, picnic tables, a hitch rail, several trailside campsites, and more secluded sites along small paths that meander into the brush. A large eucalyptus marks the path to Santa Maria Beach.

The main trail dips to cross over a small creek and, at the top of a brief incline, meets the Fire Lane Trail (5.5 miles from the trailhead). Turn right here (the Coast Trail curves left and follows the shoreline for about a mile, and then heads inland for 1.8 miles to reach the Point Reyes hostel), and climb the wide Fire Lane Trail through open coastal scrub. Look for irises in the spring, blooming among the coyote bush, ceanothus, and sticky monkeyflower. Deer frequent these hillsides, and small brush or cottontail rabbits may scurry across the trail in front of you.

After less than a mile, the trail levels and passes a small marshland, where reeds and grasses mix with the coastal scrub. You shortly reach a junction with the Laguna Trail (6.5 miles from the trailhead). Continue on the exposed route of the Fire Lane Trail. The grade is often steep, as the trail climbs several small knolls on the ascent up the ridge, but gentle descents provide respite, and great views of the coast and the Drakes Estero area offer good excuses for a rest. Before reaching the Sky Trail, the trail levels and enters a lush forest, moistened year-round by ridgetop fog drip.

At the next junction, 7.8 miles from the trailhead, turn left on the Sky Trail and follow it downhill for 0.8 mile to your starting point.

Coastal View Loop on the Bayview, Laguna, and Fire Lane trails

This trip descends the ridge on the Laguna Trail and climbs steeply back up the Fire Lane Trail. As early as February, large patches of wild iris splash the coastal scrub-covered hillsides with blue and purple flowers, and the lavender blossoms of ceanothus send a delicious fragrance into the air.

Distance: 6.1 miles
Type: Loop
Difficulty: Moderate
Facilities: None
Regulations: No bikes or dogs; horses allowed

The Bayview Trail heads north from the Sky Trailhead, roughly parallel to Limantour Road. On a gently rolling course, the narrow trail crosses mostly open vegetation of ceanothus and coyote bush, and small bishop-pine trees; in spring, iris and forget-me-nots bloom along the trailside.

After 0.7 mile, turn left at a junction with the Laguna Trail. (The Bayview Trail continues straight along the ridgecrest for 0.5 mile to the Bayview Trailhead.) Once a paved route to Laguna Ranch, the trail begins a gentle descent. Small bishop pines that reseeded after the Vision Fire line much of the trail. The blaze reinvigorated coastal scrub plants, including sticky monkeyflower, blackberry, and coyote bush. The asphalt surface of the old road

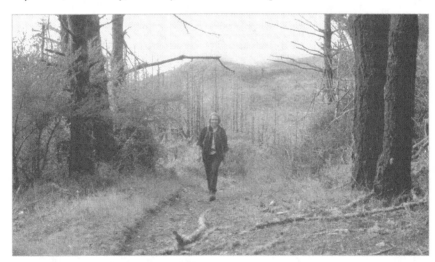

Hiker on the Fire Lane Trail

appears with frequency along the trail, reminding hikers of the ranching history of the Point Reyes peninsula.

On a mostly moderate downhill grade, with a few steeper sections, the trail descends to the former Laguna Ranch, now the site of the Point Reyes hostel and the Clem Miller Environmental Education Center. Gaps in the thick stands of bishop pines provide views to the coast and Drakes Estero. On the last descent, as the trail nears a broad meadow, willows join the trailside plants, and the shift in vegetation signals your approach to a small stream. The trail then crosses the broad meadow and reaches a short spur to the Environmental Ed center, 2 miles from the trailhead. Continue straight to cross a wooden bridge over the creek and pass a small house on your left. At 0.2 mile from the last junction, you meet the continuation of the Laguna Trail, a broad path that goes both left and right. A right takes you to the Laguna Trailhead parking area (and beyond, to the hostel). Go left to continue on the loop trip.

The trail climbs moderately through open terrain, at first on a wide grassy path, narrowing and steepening as it reaches the crest of a low hill and a junction with the Fire Lane Trail (3 miles from the trailhead). From this spot, you have views of the sweeping coastline of Drakes Bay, all the way to the point of Chimney Rock. If the expansive stretch of Limantour Beach is irresistible to you, go straight on the Fire Lane Trail to reach Coast Camp and the beach in 1 mile. Otherwise, to continue this loop, turn right and head steeply up the Fire Lane Trail.

Sensory Delights of Coastal Scrub

The aromas, colors, and textures of coastal-scrub vegetation are subtle but numerous. The intoxicating fragrance that wafts through the air along the Point Reyes trails is the result of oils that many coastal-scrub plants release. The ceanothus bushes that copiously line the trails burst with shiny green leaves, and their lavender flower clusters emit a delightful smell. The bright orange flowers of sticky monkeyflower provide color from late spring long into summer and often into fall. Iris are a special treat here, one of the first signs of spring (often appearing as early as January), in the form of large hillside clusters or single trailside blossoms.

Coyote bush produces fluffs of fuzzy white "flowers" when they go to seed in the fall. Coyote bush is a monoecious plant, meaning that the flowers on any one plant are all the same sex. (The flowers of most plants have both male and female parts—stamens and pistils, respectively.)

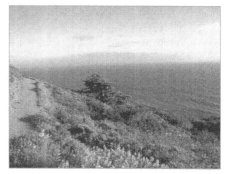

Lupine and coastal scrub along Coast Trail

The Fire Lane Trail returns to Inverness Ridge on a 2-mile, mostly exposed route. The grade is often steep, as the trail climbs several small knolls on its route, but gentle descents provide respite, and great views of the coast and the Drakes Estero area offer good excuses for a rest. Before reaching the Sky Trail, the trail levels and enters forest of Douglas-firs.

At the ridgetop junction, 5.3 miles from the trailhead, turn left on the Sky Trail and follow it downhill for 0.8 mile to your starting point.

To Limantour Beach via the Laguna and Fire Lane trails

Trip 10

From ridgetop to coast, this trip is short enough for you to enjoy an afternoon at Limantour beach. Find a friend who wants to spend a day at the beach and who will drop you at the trailhead on the way.

Distance: 5.5 miles
Type: Shuttle
Difficulty: Moderate
Facilities: Toilet, water, picnic tables, and hitch rail at Coast Camp; toilet at Limantour Beach parking lot
Regulations: No bikes or dogs; horses allowed
Driving Directions to pick-up point: This shuttle hike ends at the southern parking lot for Limantour Beach. Just before entering the main parking lot at the beach, turn left on a paved road and follow it about a half mile to its end.

The Bayview Trail heads north from the Sky Trailhead, roughly parallel to Limantour Road. The gently rolling trail crosses mostly open vegetation of ceanothus and coyote bush, and small bishop-pine trees; in spring, iris and forget-me-nots bloom along the narrow path.

Turn left at a junction with the Laguna Trail after 0.7 mile, from where the Bayview Trail continues straight along the ridgecrest for 0.5 mile to the Bayview Trailhead. Once a paved route to Laguna Ranch, the Laguna trail begins a gentle descent through a forest of small bishop pines that reseeded after the Vision Fire. The blaze reinvigorated coastal-scrub plants, including sticky monkeyflower, blackberry, and coyote bush. The asphalt surface of the old road appears with frequency along the trail, reminding hikers of the ranching history of the Point Reyes peninsula.

A few steep sections interrupt a mostly moderate downhill grade as the trail descends to the former Laguna Ranch, now the site of the Point Reyes hostel and the Clem Miller Environmental Center. You have views of the coast and of Drakes Estero through gaps in the thick stands of bishop pines. The trail nears a broad meadow where willows join the trailside plants, and the shift in vegetation signals your approach to a small stream. You then cross the meadow and reach a short spur to the Environmental Ed center, at 2 miles from the trailhead.

Continue straight to cross a wooden bridge over the creek, and pass a small house on your left. You meet the continuation of the Laguna Trail at 0.2 mile from the last junction. Go left on the broad path to continue to Limantour Beach. To reach the Laguna Trailhead parking area (and beyond, the hostel), go right. The wide grassy path narrows and steepens as it reaches the crest of a low hill and a junction with the Fire Lane Trail (3 miles from the trailhead). Go straight on the Fire Lane Trail, crossing a level section where rushes and grasses grow in a moist swale amidst the predominant coyote bush. Views take in the coastline stretching north and south. The trail soon begins to descend, rather steeply at times, and reaches the junction with the Coast Trail in 1 mile (4 miles from the trailhead).

As you walk the final half mile along the Bayview Trail, look for a ravished old live oak tree that survived the Vision Fire. If not for the vigorous new growth sprouting from its branches and roots, you might assume the tree was dead. Low-intensity and infrequent fires generally benefit oak trees, particularly evergreens like live oaks. After a fire, oaks often "crown sprout"— sending up new shoots from their upper trunk and branches.

Veer left to quickly reach Coast Camp, where a narrow path leads to the beach. Follow the smooth curve of sand northward, reaching the southern parking lot for Limantour Beach in 1.5 miles. Dip your feet in the breakers on your way up the beach and look for seals frolicking in the water on your way up the beach and whales passing by offshore. The small path to the parking lot, where your shuttle car should be waiting, is almost directly below a house that sits high on the bluff above the beach.

▶ BAYVIEW TRAILHEAD

The 1995 Vision Fire engulfed the area around the Bayview Trailhead. As it swept from Inverness Ridge to the coast, the fire left in its wake the tall trunks of burned bishop pines, but it also rejuvenated the habitat and engendered thickets of vibrant new growth and densely packed young bishop pines. The trails around the Bayview Trailhead are ideal places to observe the fascinating regeneration process of the bishop-pine forest and coastal-scrub habitats.

As of 2004, you'll be able to learn more about the role of fire in the Point Reyes ecosystem through an interpretive exhibit at the Bayview Trailhead and a trail guide for the burn area.

Driving Directions: From the Bear Valley Visitor Center, return to Bear Valley Road. Turn left and drive 1.5 miles to the Limantour Road. Turn left again and follow the road for 4.5 miles to the large gravel parking lot at the Bayview Trailhead on the east side of Limantour Road.

Facilities: None

Bayview Trail through Muddy Hollow to the Laguna Trail

Meander through dense young bishop pines and fragrant ceanothus bushes in the regenerating burn area. Take in coastal views and descend to a lush riparian environment, with excellent birdwatching opportunities. Across Limantour Road, you'll pass the hostel and the Environmental Ed Center and return to the ridgetop on the Laguna Trail.

Distance: 5 miles
Type: Loop
Difficulty: Moderate
Facilities: None
Regulations: No bikes or dogs; horses allowed

The Bayview Trail begins at the west end of the parking lot, heading toward the coast on level ground. Bishop pines seem to dominate the trailsides at first look,

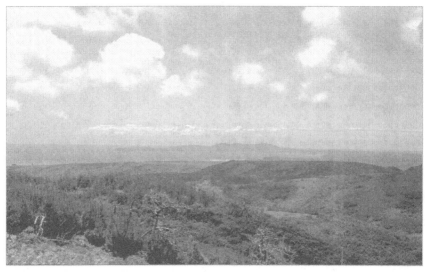

View of Drakes Bay from Bayview Trail

yet, on closer examination, surprisingly diverse vegetation joins the pines. Scattered Douglas-firs—survivors of the fire—intermingle with the pines, and huckleberry, coyote bush, and sticky monkeyflower have taken hold among the trees. As the trail begins a gentle descent, coffeeberry, currants, elderberry, wild blackberry, and wild cucumber form dense thickets. You soon come upon a north-facing slope thick with a rare manzanita, *Arctostaphylos virgata*. Like bishop pines, this manzanita depends on fire for germination. As you begin to descend into the riparian canyon, you reach a stand of bay laurel trees that extends down the hillside. Look for new sprouts around the burned bay laurels.

Across the deep stream canyon, the scrub-covered slopes rise to Inverness Ridge and Point Reyes Hill, the second highest point in the park at 1336 feet, and the site of superb panoramic views. (You can reach Point Reyes Hill and neighboring Mt. Vision, 1282 feet, via the Inverness Ridge Trail or Mt. Vision Road.)

The Maturing Forest

As you walk the trails in the Bayview area, you might wonder how this dense forest of young bishop pines will mature into a stately forest of widely spaced trees, wind-sculpted and fantastically gnarled. Look closely to see that some trees have already begun to edge out others. Root fungus, or ectomycorrhizal, plays an important role in the lives of bishop pines by extending the underground surface area of the tree and increasing its ability to compete for water and nutrients. A tree with a more developed root-fungus systems will edge out its neighbors and eventually establish itself as the lasting tree.

Other key players in thinning the forest are snags—the dead tree trunks that remain after a fire. When snags fall, they knock over young trees in their path, reducing competition for nutrients and clearing space in the understory so seedlings of other plants can take hold. Snags also provide habitats for animals, including storage facilities for woodpeckers and perches for raptors. Although essential to the natural ecosystem, snags are often called hazard trees: weakened by wind and rain, they eventually topple and can be dangerous to passing hikers.

Along the Bayview Trail, the dense bishop-pine forest is already in the process of thinning. Snags have knocked down young pines, and the wind-dispersed seeds of coyote bush have established themselves around the pines. Ceanothus, coffeeberry, elderberry, huckleberry, and currants are some of the shrubs that are prominent in the new forest. Ferns, wild cucumber, native blackberry, wax myrtle, and cow parsnip also line the trail.

As you descend more steeply, the bishop pines lose prominence and the low vegetation allows for expansive views over Drakes Bay. In spring, you'll see blue-eyed grass, buttercups, Indian paintbrush, and iris. Alder, currants, sedges, and cow parsnip grow in the stream canyon's moist soil. After 1.6 miles, you reach a junction with the Drakes View Trail, and continue straight on the Bayview Trail. You soon cross a wooden bridge and then follow an alder-lined stream for the next half mile. Notice the hillside of buckeye on your right. You meet Muddy Hollow Road at a stand of Monterey cypresses and turn left.

After crossing a creek, you arrive at Muddy Hollow Trailhead, 0.1 mile beyond. Follow the gravel road up a short hill to Limantour Road. Cross it and continue on a paved road that leads to the Point Reyes hostel. Pass the Coast Trail and the hostel, and after about one-third mile, you reach a small parking area at the Laguna Trailhead. Pick up the Laguna Trail here, and immediately branch left on it to skirt the Clem Miller Environmental Center. After a steady 1.3-mile climb flanked by ceanothus and young Douglas-firs, you reach the Bayview Trail at the ridgetop. Turn left and return 0.5 mile to your starting point at the Bayview Trailhead.

Trip 12 | Inverness Ridge to Bucklin Trail and return on the Bayview Trail

Follow Inverness Ridge to Point Reyes Hill, the second highest point in the park. Panoramic views of the peninsula accompany you down the Bucklin Trail, and birders will delight in the variety of avian fauna around Muddy Hollow. You'll return to the ridge on the Bayview Trail, abundant with wildflowers in spring and a great place to observe the effects of the Vision Fire.

Distance: 8.1 miles
Type: Loop
Difficulty: Strenuous
Facilities: None
Regulations: No bikes or dogs; horses allowed

Pass through the gate at the north edge of the parking lot and begin on the wide Inverness Ridge Trail. After a short descent you follow a nearly level trail, lined with thick coastal scrub, which has grown back with renewed vigor since the Vision Fire.

Your views extend to the east and west from the ridgetop trail. South of Tomales Bay, you can see to the creased slopes of Black Mountain, and farther to Barnabe Mountain in Samuel P. Taylor State Park. Dark, tree-filled gullies on Bolinas Ridge stand out against the golden hillsides of summer and fall. To the west, your view stretches across Muddy Hollow and Limantour to Drakes Bay and the sheltering arm of Chimney Rock.

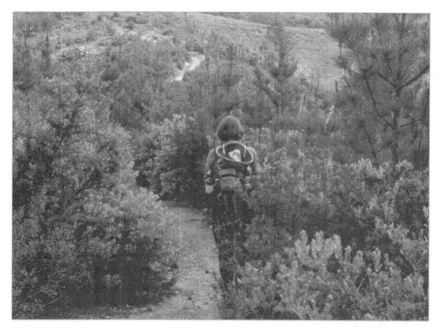

Hiker on Inverness Ridge Trail

Spring wildflowers sprout along the trail. Look for blue-eyed grass (in the iris family), delicate blue flax flowers and orange California poppies. Among bushes of ceanothus, coffeeberry, ocean spray, currant, and huckleberry, look for the peach-colored blossoms of sticky monkeyflower, big blue bunches of lupine, and pink flowers or red berries dangling from honeysuckle vines.

Seedlings and Survivors in the Forest

The Inverness Ridge Trail offers an interesting lesson in the fire resistance of different tree species. Bishop pines are highly susceptible to fire, and in fact depend on fire for survival. Their cones are sealed by a thick resin, which melts and releases the seeds only with intense heat. Once released, bishop-pine seedlings quickly germinate and thrive in the newly cleared, mineral-rich soil. Along Inverness Ridge, pre-fire bishop pines are now only stark white skeletons, charred bark peeling off, some with cones still attached to their branches.

However, several pre-fire oak, bay laurel, madrone, and Douglas-fir trees survived the fire and sprout healthy new growth. Mature Douglas-firs are fairly fire resistant, protected by their thick bark. (As young trees, Douglas-firs are very susceptible to fire.) Most of the large coniferous trees around the Bayview Trailhead are Douglas-firs, with the exception of the few rare bishop pines that survived the fire.

After about a mile, you reach a metal fire-road gate and a paved road beyond. Continue around the gate and rejoin the trail about 400 feet up the road, on the left. Now on a narrow path, you climb briefly through drier terrain. Tightly packed young bishop pines line the trail, along with manzanita, huckleberry, and ceanothus bushes. Pass the Drakes View Trail (1.4 miles from the trailhead) and continue along Inverness Ridge. You soon descend to a notch in the ridge, where you have spectacular views east across Tomales Bay and west over the coastal slopes to the ocean.

You now climb a couple of gradual switchbacks up the flank of Point Reyes Hill on a narrow, grass-lined trail. In less than a mile, you reach the 1336-foot highpoint and some fenced-off spherical structures, property of the Federal Aviation Administration. They house a directional signal that guides planes to the San Francisco Airport.

At the summit (2.8 miles from the trailhead), follow the paved road for about 50 yards to find the Bucklin Trail on the left. The trail descends the open coastal slope for 2.4 miles, among low stands of coyote bush and lupine and through dense tunnels of bishop pine and ceanothus. Look for spring wildflowers, including blue-eyed grass, suncups, iris, Indian paintbrush, and the rare pussy ears lily (*Calochortus tolmei*). You have spectacular views of the Drakes and Limantour esteros, the headlands, and the Great Beach.

At the junction of Muddy Hollow Road and the Bucklin Trail, you are on the margin of the Phillip Burton Wilderness Area and functioning ranchlands. To the right, the road leaves the wilderness area and reaches Home Ranch, where the Shafter dairy empire that commandeered much of Point Reyes in the second half of the 1800s was headquartered. Still intact today, Home Ranch (also called Murphy Ranch) now raises beef cattle.

Although grazing is not permitted in the designated wilderness, the Muddy Hollow area was once "cow heaven," as the ranch owners called it. The Steele family ranch occupied these hillsides and was well-known for its high-quality butter and cheese. As you near the Bayview Trail, you'll see a stand of Monterey cypress on the original ranch site.

Turn left on Muddy Hollow Road, follow its nearly level course for 0.8 mile to the Bayview Trail, and turn left again. The Bayview Trail is level as it follows the course of a creek. After passing the Drakes View Trail (an alternative route to the trailhead that would add about 1.3 miles to your trip), you begin a steady but gradual climb. The slope eases before you reach the trailhead, and the final half mile or so is a nearly level trail through dense bishop pines, ceanothus, currants, and coyote bush. (See the first part of Trip 11 for a detailed description, in reverse, of this segment of the Bayview Trail.)

The Muddy Hollow trailhead used to afford excellent loop trips around Limantour Estero and surrounding highlands. Since the Muddy Hollow Trail has become indistinguishable from the creekbed it paralleled (aptly reflecting its name), the trail has been closed, eliminating most loops in this area except those that head east up the ridge (on the Drakes View, Bucklin, and Bayview trails— see trips from the Bayview Trailhead). Little-traveled but rich in history, wildlife, and beauty, the Muddy Hollow area deserves exploration.

Driving Directions: From the Bear Valley Visitor Center, return to Bear Valley Road. Turn left and drive 1.5 miles to the Limantour Road. Turn left again, follow the road for 6 miles, and turn right on the gravel road to Muddy Hollow. The trailhead parking lot is 0.1 mile beyond.

Facilities: None

Muddy Hollow Road

Trip 13

Combine a day at Limantour Beach with a short walk along this old ranch road. Cypress trees mark the site of one of the peninsula's first dairy ranches, Muddy Hollow Ranch. A short walk on Muddy Hollow Road connects to the Glenbrook Trail, which you can follow for nearly 4 miles (but you'll have to retrace your steps to return).

Distance: 3 miles round trip to Glenbrook Trail
Type: Out-and-back
Difficulty: Easy
Facilities: None
Regulations: No bikes or dogs.

After passing through a gate at the trailhead, you arrive at a stream where recent restoration work is improving fish habitat. Jump across the stream to reach a large stand of Monterey cypress trees that marks the site of one of the peninsula's first dairy ranches. From the trees, the Bayview Trail branches right to reach the Bayview Trailhead on Inverness Ridge, and you continue straight on Muddy Hollow Road between low coastal hills. The coyote bush that covers these hillsides was partner to the eventual downfall of the dairy industry here—grazing could not keep the hearty brush at bay. In spring, large clumps of blue-purple iris color the slopes, and since the Vision Fire of 1995, hundreds of small bishop pines have appeared among the coyote bushes.

From the Bayview Trail junction, Muddy Hollow Road ascends gently to the crest of a small rise, where you see two small ponds to the west, built by ranchers in the 1950s as watering holes for cattle. Developers who had their eye on this area figured the ponds into their plans for a subdivisions. Today, the ponds are habitat for endangered red-legged frogs.

After 0.9 mile from the trailhead, you pass the Bucklin Trail, another route to Inverness Ridge. Continue on the road, shortly reaching the creek drainage of Glenbrook Creek. Beyond, the Glenbrook Trail branches right (1.5 miles from the trailhead). Turn here to follow the trail across open moors for up to 4 miles, or turn around and head back to the Muddy Hollow Trailhead.

Evolution of a Road

Coast Miwok probably first established the route of Muddy Hollow Road. Historians believe Sir Francis Drake's party then followed it in 1579, and later ranchers and settlers on the peninsula used the route to reach Olema. Ranch owners widened and realigned the road in the 1950s, making the eroded cuts you can see alongside. In the 1960s and 1970s, Muddy Hollow Road was the proposed route from Limantour Road to the lighthouse on the point, but a strong public outcry thwarted the plans.

►LAGUNA TRAILHEAD

The trailheads along the hostel access road provide excellent access to the coast on relatively flat trails. Bikes are allowed on the Coast Trail from the trailhead to Coast Camp

Driving Directions: From the Bear Valley Visitor Center, return to Bear Valley Road. Turn left and drive 1.5 miles to the Limantour Road. Turn left again, follow the road for 6 miles, and turn left onto Laguna Road. (The short road to the Muddy Hollow trailhead is on your right.) The Coast Trail begins just across the road from the Point Reyes hostel; parking is available on the side of the road. The Laguna Trail begins 0.3 mile farther down the road, and the Clem Miller Environmental Education Center is at the end of the road.

Facilities: No water or restrooms; Environmental Ed Center facilities are available by group reservation only.

The Point Reyes hostel stands on the site of the Laguna Ranch, one of the premier dairy ranches on the Point Reyes peninsula. The U.S. Army leased the land during World War II and built roads, barracks, and gun emplacements. After the war, Laguna Ranch reverted to a dairy and beef ranch, and the new owner planted a garden with over 100 varieties of lilies and daffodils. The bright flowers still blossom every spring near the hostel. The National Park Service bought the property in 1971 and converted the buildings into the hostel and park residences. You can visit the hostel after 4:30 P.M., or spend the night there (see page 94 for details).

Laguna–Fire Lane–Coast Trail Loop

This gentle hike follows wide trails through low chaparral and along coastal dunes, and offers outstanding vistas of Drakes Bay and Chimney Rock. Visit the beach at Coast Camp or extend the hike by continuing a mile beyond the camp to fantastic Sculptured Beach. Look for deer grazing in the scrub and rabbits scurrying across the trail.

Distance: 4.9 miles
Type: Loop
Difficulty: Easy
Facilities: Toilet, water, picnic tables at Coast Camp

Park in the dirt parking lot at the Laguna Trailhead just beyond the Point Reyes hostel and begin on the Laguna Trail. A gradual climb takes you up the rutted and grassy trail, where you'll likely encounter some muddy spots in winter. You crest a low rise after 0.8 mile and arrive at a junction with the Fire Lane Trail, where you have your first views of the coast. The Laguna Trail ends here and you continue south (seemingly west, but the water actually lies to the south here, because of the angle of the land and the bay) on the Fire Lane Trail for 1 mile to Coast Camp. The trail is at first level and then it gently descends, flanked by coyote bush and ceanothus, thicker and more vigorous than ever since the 1995 fire.

When you reach the Coast Trail, go left to reach Coast Camp in 0.1 mile. You pass an access trail to several campsites on the hill above the camp, and at

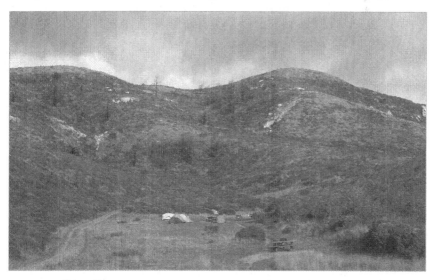

Coast Camp

the northern edge of the camp a small path leads to the beach, past the large eucalyptus that marks the camp's location from a great distance away. Water, toilets, picnic tables, grills, and a hitch rail are available at the camp.

Side Trip to Sculptured Beach

A brief jaunt (1.1 miles round trip) south along the Coast Trail brings you to a short path marked by a small sign among ceanothus bushes. The path descends to Sculptured Beach, where eroding ochre cliffs form contoured canyons behind the sand. Complexly layered rocks provide sites for tidepools. At low tide, you can go north on the beach to Coast Camp, and rejoin the described hike there. At *really* low tide (minus), you can go south along the beach to visit Secret Beach.

To return to the trailhead, retrace your steps to the Fire Lane/Coast trails junction and follow the wide and smooth Coast Trail north along the coastline for about 1 mile. The Limantour dunes obscure your view of the immediate coast, but you can look ahead to the wide sweep of Drakes Bay. Be sure to turn around also and take in views of the slopes of Inverness Ridge and the southern line of the coast. The trail leads inland after about a mile and passes a small marsh, circled by cattails, tules, and willows.

You saunter alongside a small creek for the next 1.7 miles, where alders grow densely along the bank. The deciduous alders lose their leaves in fall and delicate cones hang from the branches. When you reach the trailhead at the hostel, go right and follow the paved road for 0.3 mile to your starting point at the Laguna Trailhead.

►LIMANTOUR BEACH AND TRAILHEAD

Long walks, wading, and wildlife-viewing: Limantour Beach and Estero are a popular weekend destination for families, picnickers, and naturalists. Leashed dogs are allowed on the southern end of the beach.

Beach Grasses and Dune Ecology

The coarse grasses that cover the sandy mounds behind Limantour are European beach grass (*Ammphila arenaria*), first introduced to the Pacific Coast in Golden Gate Park in the 1890s to stabilize the dunes. The nonnative grass quickly took over the American dune grass (*Elymus mollis*), permanently altering the environment: it allows few other plant species to grow and restricts the burrowing places of animals, thus reducing the diversity of both plants and animals in the dunes. One hearty native plant, dune lupine (*Lupinus chamissonis*), however, grows in ubiquitous clumps behind Limantour Beach. Another vigorous plant, a small-leaved, ground-hugging variety of coyote bush, also defies the beach grass.

Driving Directions: From the Bear Valley Visitor Center, return to Bear Valley Road. Turn left and drive 1.5 miles to the Limantour Road. Turn left again and follow the road for 7.5 miles to its end at a large parking lot. Just before the lot, you can turn left on a road that leads a half mile to a smaller parking lot also with beach access.

Facilities: Toilets, water, and phone near main parking lot; toilet at secondary lot

Regulations: No dogs west of the trail from the parking area; dogs on leash allowed east of the trail; no camping; no fires

The Beach: Located relatively close to Bear Valley, Limantour may well be the most-visited beach in the seashore, but it is also one of the most idyllic. Grass-covered dunes ripple behind the broad strip of sand, part of the 8-mile sweep of Drakes Bay coastline.

Beach-goers have many activity options at Limantour. Wildlife-watchers will enjoy the bird-rich marshlands and tidal waters of Limantour Estero and the harbor seal population on the spit; the long stretch of clean, soft sand makes for great beach walks. Hikers can climb to the ridgetop or follow the Coast Trail south on the bluffs. And brave swimmers will find the protected waters of Drakes Bay welcoming (although no lifeguard is on duty and the strong currents make the water potentially dangerous for swimming).

Drakes Beach Estates—Almost

Priceless real estate or habitat for pelicans, harbor seals, and lupine? As hard as it is to imagine today, the dunes behind Limantour were close to becoming subdivisions of half-acre homesites, with a beach club, golf course, boat harbor, and commercial shops. In the 1950s, developers planned Drakes Beach Estates and, racing against the planned national seashore, began work on a road from Inverness Ridge to the site. Advertisements in the *San Rafael Independent Journal* encouraged buyers to move quickly: "Option your Drakes Bay lot now!" Developers built 18 homes before the National Park Service acquired the land.

Congress Near Adjournment—Option Your Drake's Bay Lot Now!

You can put a "hold" on a fabulous Drake's Bay homesite until you're SURE it will remain private property!

Despite years of threats and thunderous publicity, the Point Reyes National Seashore bill has NOT YET PASSED—and Congress adjourns in not too many weeks.

Drake's Bay Unit No. 2 JUST RECORDED. Dramatic view lots overlooking the deep blue Bay and the beautiful White Cliffs of Point Reyes. The "find" of a lifetime!

BE SAFE—Option your lot now . . . complete your purchase after the "National Seashore" washes away!

From $5,500 . . . Attractive Terms

DRAKE'S BAY ESTATES, INC.

Phone: 453-6630 • 453-4280

National Park Service

1950s newspaper advertisement

Beach Walk to Coast Camp

Trip 15

A simple stroll down Limantour Beach follows the curve of Drakes Bay to reach Coast Camp. At low tide, you can explore Sculptured and Secret beaches beyond.

Distance: 2.8 miles round trip to Coast Camp
Type: Out-and-back
Difficulty: Easy
Facilities: Toilets, water, and phone at the trailhead; toilets and water at Coast Camp
Regulations: Dogs on leash allowed east of the trail from the parking area. No bikes.

HARBOR SEALS: DO NOT DISTURB

Gathered on sandy spits and tidal mudflats, harbor seals look like small, sausage-shaped lumps. Their round bodies range in color from silvery to brown or black and are also spotted. Some have a reddish sheen to their fur, which may be an accumulation of iron on the hair shafts. Harbor seals have short necks and small hind flippers, and since they can't rotate their pelvis to use their rear flippers for walking, they rarely stray far from water. But like humans, harbor seals need sleep and rest. Every day, after feeding at night, they "haul out" on land and spend low-tide periods resting and absorbing heat from the sun.

You can usually see harbor seal pups at Point Reyes between March and June. The best places to see them are the sandbars at the tip of Limantour Spit and around Drakes Estero. But don't get too close! Extremely alert animals, harbor seals watch human activity with curiosity and are very sensitive to disturbance—from humans, dogs, boats, airplanes and even other wild animals. Merely by passing a haul-out in a quiet kayak, you might cause the seals to "flush"—make a mass exodus from their sandy spit into the water. Flushing disrupts seals' essential resting time and often separates pups from their mothers. Repeated disturbances at a particular site can reduce reproduction rates and cause the seals to permanently abandon a particular haul-out site.

The area encompassed by Point Reyes National Seashore and the Gulf of the Farallones National Marine Sanctuary supports the largest concentration of harbor seals on mainland California, about 20 percent of the state population. Both agencies conduct volunteer programs that monitor the affect of human activity

Begin on the small trail from the secondary parking lot at Limantour Beach. Mark the location of the lot for your return by the house on the hillside above. Follow the path to the beach and then head south (left) along the sand. Look for seals playing in the waters and for whales passing by in winter and spring.

A large eucalyptus tree on the bluff marks Coast Camp, 1.4 miles down the beach. As you near the camp, the cliffs beyond the sand gain height and prominence, and host a number of delightful plants. Leave the shoreline to get a closer look: strands of morning glory trail across the cliff faces, and small clusters of dudleya grow on the eroding walls, along with orange sticky monkeyflower, yellow lizard tail, and blue lupine. In small, damp crevices, ferns and seep monkeyflowers take advantage of the moisture.

Beyond Coast Camp, at low tide you can continue along the sand to Sculptured Beach. (See page 71 about Sculptured Beach.) In the winter, waves often wash away the sand, exposing layered terraces of rock. In summer, the sandy beach is easier to walk on and explore tidepools.

on harbor seal populations, and work together to minimize disturbance to harbor seals.

Please follow these guidelines when you find yourself near seals:
• The Marine Mammal Act recommends that you stay at least 300 feet from harbor seals, on land or in the water. If you notice that your presence causes the seals to raise their heads, move away immediately. Use binoculars! If you get too close and flush the animals into the water, you won't see them anyway.
• Do not touch or attempt to move lone animals. Adults may leave their pups alone when they forage.
• Respect closures to certain areas during breeding season, March 15 to June 30. Drakes Estero is closed to boating but hiking is permitted. Tomales Point and Limantour Spit remain open, but signs are posted to caution against disturbance.

Check out www.watchablewildlife.org for further guidelines on paddlers' etiquette for responsible wildlife viewing.

Harbor Seal or Sea Lion?

People often confuse harbor seals and sea lions, but if you know what to look for, you can easily tell the two species apart. Harbor seals are smaller than adult sea lions, are generally lighter in color, and have spots. Since seals can't rotate their pelvis, they can't waddle or walk on land, and they stick close to water. Sea lions, on the other hand, use their back flippers to move themselves about with agility. Another important difference is that harbor seals don't have external ear flaps like sea lions do.

Limantour Spit Trail

Limantour Spit is an easy but invigorating walk along the dunes between Limantour Estero and Beach. On clear days you'll have stunning views north of Chimney Rock and Drakes Head, and south along the coast and up Inverness Ridge. Look for shorebirds in the estero and harbor seals on the spit.

Distance: 2 miles round trip on trail (you can continue on the beach for about 2 miles beyond the trail's end)
Type: Out-and-back
Difficulty: Easy
Facilities: Toilets, water, and phone at the trailhead
Regulations: No dogs, bikes, or horses

Begin on the trail to the beach from the main parking lot. Past the wooden walkway through the marsh, turn right on a small path that heads across the dunes behind the beach. On a narrow strip of land between Limantour Estero and Beach, the trail follows the route of an old road that led to the planned development of Drakes Beach Estates. Much earlier, Coast Miwok inhabited the area around Limantour Estero, and archeologists have discovered middens containing bones, shells, baskets, and old tools.

Shorebirds are most abundant at Limantour Estero from October through March, when they gather to feast on the abundance of food in the tidal waters. You might see the turned-up tail of the marsh wren, a small, insect-eating bird that perches among reeds and grasses in marshy areas along the spit trail. From late spring into early fall, you'll likely see brown pelicans, who often roost on the spit and forage for fish at Limantour Beach.

Clumps of lupine, dwarf coyote bush, and beach grass (which stings your thighs as you brush past) cover the dunes. Freshwater streams and salty ocean water both empty into Limantour Estero, creating a brackish habitat that supports a diverse array of plants and animals. Saltwater plants like pickleweed grow in close range of freshwater species like silverweed.

The dunes diminish in height as you continue, grasses and lupine grow closer together on rumpled mounds of sand, and the trail becomes harder to follow. Breaks in the dunes, where high tide can wash freely between the estero and the ocean, appear more frequently. The trail ends after about a mile, and you can continue on the beach to the far end of the spit.

SIR FRANCIS DRAKE HIGHWAY TRAILS AND BEACHES

*"[The lighthouse road] was a wretched road, and crawling
wagons sank to their axles in the winter's mud. Children riding their carts to the school...pulled aside to let the drover
and his hogs go by. Hogs were everywhere, clogging the road."*
—Jack Mason, *Point Reyes: The Solemn Land*

Sir Francis Drake Highway descends from Inverness Ridge to the lowlands of
Drakes Estero and sets off across the rolling pasturelands and inland-stretching
dunes of the outer point. You may feel as though you are leaving the populated
world behind, especially when the fog hangs low over the land. Yet, en route,
you'll pass several dairy ranches that have operated on the peninsula since the
19th century, many in the same family for generations.

As the road dips into a broad level plain beyond Drakes Estero, you'll notice
a row of Monterey cypress on the right. The tall, straight trees mark the road to
the former Radio Corporation of America (RCA) facility. Point Reyes' long
extension into the Pacific Ocean makes it an ideal location for radio transmis-
sion. In 1929, RCA bought G Ranch and moved its Tomales Bay station here.
Amelia Earhart's final transmissions came through this station, as did important
communications from the Pacific during World War II.

The road ends at Point Reyes itself, where a lighthouse warns ships of the
rocky tip of land that juts into the Pacific. The 11-mile Point Reyes Beach
stretches north from the point, exposed to strong winds and heavy surf. To the
south, Drakes Bay is protected by the point. Plan on a 45-minute drive from
Bear Valley to the lighthouse.

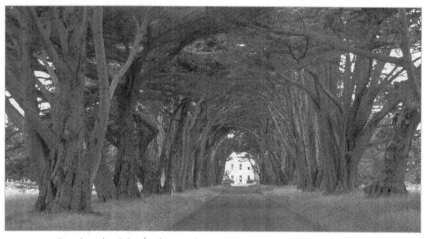

Road to the RCA facility on the outer point

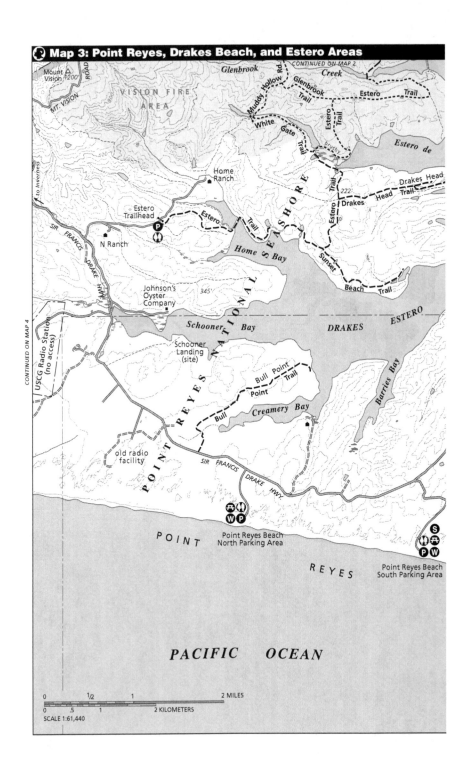

Mount
Vision 1200'

VISION FIRE
AREA

MT. VISION

ROAD

Glenbrook

CONTINUED ON MAP 2

Creek

Muddy Hollow Rd.

Glenbrook
Trail

Estero   Trail

Estero
Trail

White   Gate
Trail

Estero   Trail

Estero de

to Inverness

SIR   FRANCIS   DRAKE   HWY.

Home
Ranch

Estero
Trailhead

P

N Ranch

Estero   Trail

Home Bay

Drakes Head

Estero Trail

222'

Drakes
Head Trail

Drakes

NATIONAL   SEASHORE

Johnson's
Oyster
Company

345'

Sunset

Beach   Trail

CONTINUED ON MAP 4

USCG Radio Station
(no access)

Schooner   Bay

DRAKES   ESTERO

Schooner
Landing
(site)

POINT   REYES

Bull Point   Trail

Point

Bull

Creamery Bay

Barries Bay

old radio
facility

SIR   FRANCIS   DRAKE   HWY.

P

W   P

Point Reyes Beach
North Parking Area

S

P
W

POINT

REYES

Point Reyes Beach
South Parking Area

PACIFIC   OCEAN

0   1/2   1   2 MILES
0   .5   1   2 KILOMETERS
SCALE 1:61,440

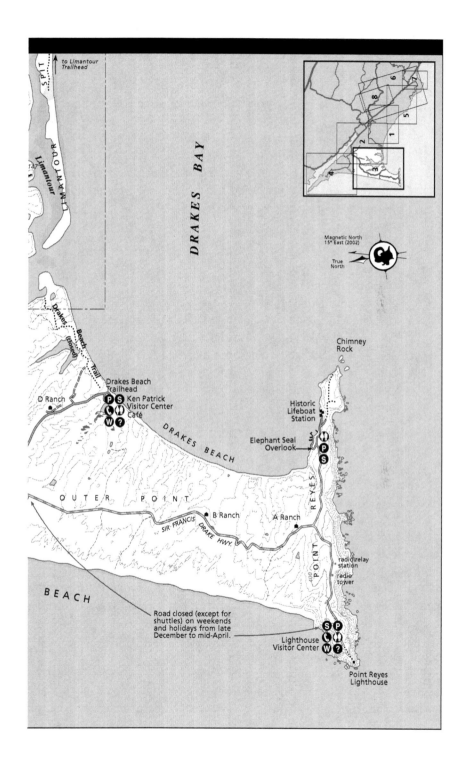

to Limantour
Trailhead

LIMANTOUR SPIT

Limantour

DRAKES BAY

Magnetic North
15° East (2002)

True
North

Chimney
Rock

Drakes
Beach
Trail (closed)

Drakes Beach
Trailhead

D Ranch

Ken Patrick
Visitor Center

Café

P S
L M
W ?

Historic
Lifeboat
Station

Elephant Seal
Overlook

P
P
S

DRAKES BEACH

OUTER   POINT

SIR FRANCIS DRAKE HWY.

B Ranch

A Ranch

POINT   REYES

radio relay
station

radio
tower

400

BEACH

Road closed (except for
shuttles) on weekends
and holidays from late
December to mid-April.

Lighthouse
Visitor Center

S P
L M
W ?

Point Reyes
Lighthouse

Drive to Point Reyes Hill and Mt. Vision

For those who want to experience dramatic vistas at Point Reyes without exerting themselves, the road from Sir Francis Drake Highway to Mt. Vision provides just the opportunity. Views improve with every curve on this 3-mile trip up the narrow and twisting Mt. Vision Road. From the road-end, you can walk a short distance to Point Reyes Hill, where the Inverness Ridge and the Bucklin trails offer possibilities of short strolls or longer loop hikes.

Distance: 3 miles from Sir Francis Drake Highway to end of road at Mt. Vision

Type: Out-and-back drive

Facilities: None

Regulations: No dogs on trails

Driving Directions: From the Bear Valley Visitor Center, return to Bear Valley Road and turn left. In 2 miles, turn left again on Sir Francis Drake Highway and continue through Inverness to the junction with Pierce Point Road (2.5 miles past Inverness). Bear left to stay on Sir Francis Drake, and 1 mile beyond the junction turn left on Mt. Vision Road.

The narrow, serpentine Mt. Vision Road winds up the hillside for 3 miles, and ooos and ahhhs over the expanding view increase with each turn. At the summit (1282'), panoramic views of the countryside greet you: on clear days, you'll see the entire Point Reyes peninsula, the coast as it stretches north and south, plus the peaks of Mts. St. Helena, Diablo, and Tamalpais. A gate bars the road beyond Mt. Vision, but you can continue on foot to nearby Point Reyes Hill, the second highest point on the peninsula at 1336 feet (after Mt. Wittenberg).

The fenced-off spherical structures near the summit of Point Reyes Hill are property of the Federal Aviation Administration. They house a directional signal that guides planes to the San Francisco Airport. At the summit, the Inverness Ridge Trail goes south on a 2.8-mile, view-filled trip to the Bayview Trailhead, and the Bucklin Trail descends to Muddy Hollow Road. (A 7- or 8-mile loop trip follows the Bucklin Trail to Muddy Hollow Road and returns via the Bayview or Drakes View trail. See Trip 12.)

The 1995 fire that burned over 12,000 acres in the seashore started on the western slope of Mt. Vision, and quickly engulfed the mountain, burning intensely in the bishop-pine forest. This area is now an excellent place to marvel at the regenerative capacities of the ecosystem. In spring, a short walk from your car will reveal a profusion of roadside wildflowers, including the ubiquitous poppy and lupine, but also seaside daisy, baby blue eyes, and harvest brodiaea.

Estero Trail to Drakes Head

Excellent bird-watching in the estero, the largest harbor seal breeding colony at Point Reyes, abundant iris in the spring, and outstanding views from Drakes Head make this a great all-around hike or bike ride. The trail leads over gently rolling moors above Home Bay on Drakes Estero and then crosses open pastureland to reach Drakes Head. You're in grazing country here—outside of the seashore's designated wilderness area—so in addition to the wildlife, you'll see plenty of patches of cow dung, but the view from Drakes Head is well worth it.

Distance: 2 miles round trip to bridge and viewing spot; 9.4 miles round trip to Drakes Head
First 0.5 mile wheelchair-accessible
Type: Out-and-back
Difficulty: Strenuous
Facilities: Toilets at trailhead; no water
Regulations: Bikes and horses allowed; no dogs
Driving directions: From the Bear Valley Visitor Center, return to Bear Valley Road and turn left. In 2 miles, turn left again on Sir Francis Drake Highway and continue through Inverness to the junction with Pierce Point Road (2.5 miles past Inverness). Bear left to stay on Sir Francis Drake, and about 2 miles beyond the junction turn left on a road signed to ESTERO TRAILHEAD; the trailhead is about a half mile farther.

Inverness Ridge is a dramatic backdrop to these low tidal moors. From the trailhead you can see Mt. Vision, Point Reyes Hill, and Mt. Wittenberg, the high points along the ridge. The trail sets out toward the estero on a level course. The first half mile is wheelchair-accessible, although some muddy patches may be difficult in wet months. The trail soon begins a gentle descent through a former Christmas tree farm, an odd patch of trees in an otherwise open landscape. Look for owls perched on the branches of Monterey pines.

You reach the shores of the upper estero after about a mile and cross a narrow inlet of Home Bay on a bridge. A weathered sign at the water's edge warns against approaching seal pups; mothers abandon their young if they have been touched by humans. The bridge offers a good vantage point to pause and look for birds, especially during low tide when crabs and worms in the mudflats attract herons, egrets, and other shorebirds. Also watch for hawks as they glide over the grasslands in search of small rodents.

Now on the southwest side of Home Bay, the trail ascends gradually to reach a knoll high above the estero. Coyote bush, lupine, currant, blackberry, sticky monkeyflower, and ceanothus are among the trailside plants. In late winter and spring, low clumps of blue iris flowers dot the grasslands. Cows graze these grasslands, so expect to see evidence of the friendly animals. In the next mile or so, you make a couple of roller-coaster ascents and descents and pass through two cattle stiles. A large eucalyptus atop a hill makes a good spot to take a break and appreciate views across the estero.

After 2.6 miles, you reach a junction with the Sunset Beach Trail, which continues along Drakes Estero for another 1.4 miles and then peters out in a bramble of poison oak, blackberry, and coyote bush.

To reach Drakes Head, turn left and follow the Estero Trail up a gentle rise and across open pastureland. Cow paths and ranch roads branch off in various

FROM BUSTLING PORT TO WILDLIFE HAVEN

Estero is the Spanish word for estuary, a brackish body of water that supports both fresh- and saltwater species. At Drakes Estero, plants like pickleweed and saltgrass grow near the coast in the saline tidal marshlands. Freshwater plants grow near creek inlets at the head of the marsh. The estero's varied habitats make it one of the prime wildlife-viewing areas on the peninsula, home to landbirds, shorebirds, and seabirds.

Shorebirds feast on the wealth of invertebrates that live in the tidal flats and sandy beaches around esteros. Brown and white pelicans visit the sand bars at the mouth of the estero. Look for brown pelicans during the non-breeding season, from May or June through December; white pelicans arrive in August and stay through January. Herons, egrets, black brants, willets, and godwits also frequent the estero, and you may see an owl or two in the Monterey pines along the trail. Seals often haul-out on sandbars near the mouth of the estero. They are easily disturbed by humans, so bring binoculars and watch them from a distance.

Today a haven for birds and harbor seals, Drakes Estero was once bustling with boats on trips to and from San Francisco. During the height of the Point Reyes dairying days, the bay was a navigable waterway and served as the main access to San Francisco markets. Schooners left from the 200-foot-long pier on Schooner Bay, loaded with precious Point Reyes butter and hogs for merchants and slaughterhouses in the city, and returned with feed for animals. Larger boats brought redwood planks from Santa Cruz forests, used as building material for barns and farmhouses.

You can see Home Ranch (also called Murphy Ranch), one of the oldest operating ranches in Point Reyes today, from the Drakes Estero Trailhead. In its heyday, some 300 cows and 20 or more whitewashed buildings, including a butcher shop and a blacksmith shop, comprised the 2500-acre ranch. The historic ranch narrowly escaped the Vision Fire of 1995.

directions, so follow the blue and white arrows to stay on track. You pass through a cattle stile after 0.7 mile and go right to pick up the Drakes Head Trail. The 1.4-mile trail dwindles into a rutted path as it heads southwest toward the ocean. Press on, for whatever discouragement you feel will dissipate at first glimpse of the view from Drakes Head.

Before reaching a clump of trees that marks the site of the former Drakes Head Ranch, you branch right and climb a small rise to reach the head. The high bluff commands a sweeping view of the peninsula. On clear days you'll see Chimney Rock to the north; Limantour Spit and Estero adjacent to you; and beyond, to the south, Limantour Beach, Arch Rock, Wildcat Beach, and Double Point. Clear days afford views past the Golden Gate to Montara Mountain near Half Moon Bay. Look inland for views of Drakes Estero and the broad coastal plain as it rises toward Inverness Ridge. When you're ready to return, retrace your steps to the trailhead.

Ranching on Drakes Head

Drakes Head Ranch began as a dairy ranch, but in the 1920s and 1930s, as the dairy industry at Point Reyes struggled, it converted to a vegetable farm. A group of Italian farmers grew artichokes and Japanese farmers cultivated peas. When World War II broke out, the Japanese were forced into interment camps and a law prohibited Italians from being within a certain distance of the coast. In the Point Reyes area, Italians were not allowed west of Highway 1. The ranch was abandoned completely by the mid-1950s, and the National Park Service later demolished the buildings.

Bull Point Trail

Trip 19

This level stroll on an old farm road heads across the open grasslands of the outer point to the shores of Drakes Estero. You're likely to see many migratory birds in the estero, and seals and sea lions often gather on the beach at the trail's end.

Distance: 3.8 miles round trip
Type: Out-and-back
Difficulty: Easy
Facilities: No water or toilets.
Regulations: No bikes, horses, or dogs
Driving directions: From the Bear Valley Visitor Center, return to Bear Valley Road and turn left. In 2 miles, turn left again on Sir Francis Drake Highway and continue through Inverness to the junction with Pierce Point Road (2.5 miles past Inverness). Bear left to

stay on Sir Francis Drake, and 4.8 miles past the junction turn left into a small gravel parking lot.

Shortly after starting out across the grasslands, you skirt the remnants of Historic F Ranch—marked only by a few old cypress and eucalyptus trees. F Ranch was once a busy outpost with a landing on Schooner Bay, the biggest barn on the point, and a post office run by the ranchers and their wives. The trail continues overland and gently climbs to a knoll above Creamery Bay, an arm of Drakes Estero. Cows graze among the clumps of dwarf coyote bush and lupine that cover the grasslands. You have expansive views across the moors to Inverness Ridge, capped by Point Reyes Hill, Mt. Vision, and Mt. Wittenberg. The broad mouth of the bay gapes directly ahead of you, enclosed by Chimney Rock to the north and Limantour Spit to the south.

After almost 2 miles the trail reaches the eroding cliffs above Drakes Estero, where a few trees grow precariously in the loose soil. Look for pelicans, egrets, black brant, and other migratory birds. Schooner Bay reaches inland to your left, and the Estero Trail traces the shores of Home Bay beyond.

▶ DRAKES BEACH

Something for everyone—beach walkers, waders, geology and history buffs, wildlife-scouts—plus a visitor center and cafe.

Driving Directions: From the Bear Valley Visitor Center, return to Bear Valley Road and turn left. In 2 miles, turn left again on Sir Francis Drake Highway and continue through Inverness to the junction with Pierce Point Road (2.5 miles past Inverness). Bear left to stay on Sir Francis Drake, and 7.5 miles past the junction turn left on a road signed for DRAKES BEACH and follow it to the large parking lot. **Facilities:** Water, restrooms and dressing rooms, shower, picnic tables, grills, cafe, and visitor center

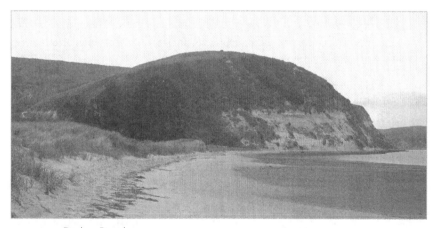

Drakes Beach

Regulations: No dogs

In 1938, the area around Drakes Beach became the first public holding in what is now Point Reyes National Seashore. A group of private citizens bought a 52-acre parcel of land behind Drakes Beach and turned it over to Marin County for public use as a beach, park, and recreation area. It subsequently became part of the national seashore.

Ken Patrick Visitor Center

The visitor center at Drakes Beach, aside from providing a warm escape on cold days, furnishes displays on maritime history and the marine environment. It's an excellent place to learn the controversial and intriguing story of Sir Francis Drake. A 200-gallon aquarium houses aquatic life from Drakes Bay, and you can view a minke-whale skeleton and other natural history exhibits.

Hours: Open weekends and holidays from 10 A.M. to 5 P.M.; closed December 25. Wheelchair-accessible.

Drakes Beach Cafe

Known for their clam chowder and oyster stew, Drakes Beach Cafe offers tasty meals and snacks with a view you can't beat. Weather permitting, you can sit indoors or out.

Shuttle Service from Drakes Beach

On weekends and holidays from late December through mid-April, Sir Francis Drake Highway is closed at South Beach. A shuttle-bus service leaves from the Drakes Beach parking lot and takes visitors to the lighthouse and Chimney Rock. Reservations are not required. Adult tickets cost $5; children 12 and under ride free.

The Beach: Drakes Beach is a delightful combination of well-used recreation area and spectacular and solitary natural beauty, abutted by working ranchland. To enjoy it, come prepared with warm clothes even when the sun is shining at Bear Valley, and bundle up for a stroll down the beach or a picnic. The outer point is known for dense fogs and bone-chilling cold, and Drakes Beach, although more protected than Pacific beaches, is no exception. The sun does shine at Drakes Beach, although more often in winter than in summer. Sunny weekends in February bring out surfers riding the feeble swells, picnickers enjoying the winter sun, beach-loafers in bathing suits, and a few brave swimmers and waders.

In any weather, on just a short walk down the beach, you can leave behind the crowds near the visitor center and immediate beachfront. Head south along the beach to look for one of the Drake monuments and to reach the mouth of Drakes Estero. The sand on the beach shifts with the seasons and the tides, sometimes exposing rocky shelves which you'll have to climb over at high tide.

When fog obscures the sweep of the beach that extends south toward Limantour, your world reduces to the bay and the cliffs that rise to the rolling pastureland above. The only sounds you'll hear are the crashing of the waves and the continuous process of erosion as small pebbles trickle down the cliffs.

After about half a mile on the beach, the cliffs give way to a large horseshoe-shaped pond, just behind the dunes. Tide permitting, continue down the beach to the mouth of Drakes Estero, about another half a mile ahead. A weathered post on the dunes bears a plaque that marks this as Drake's landing site.

The cream-colored cliffs that backdrop the bay are composed of a marine sediment called the Drakes Bay Formation. Greensand lies at the base of the formation and contains fossilized bones of fish, seals, and whales, as well as invertebrates. Covering the greensand is shale, which is in turn overlain by siltstones and mudstones. The softness of these uppermost sediments is responsible for the erosion you can see taking place by the minute.

Beyond the dunes, a shallow channel connects Drakes Estero to the ocean. Schooners entered here in the 1800s to pick up butter from the landing in the estero. Harbor seals often haul out on the mudflats near the mouth of the estero. Being careful not to disturb them, you can circle the dunes and follow the shoreline of the estero inland. A stand of Monterey cypress near the bluff houses several heron nests. Instead of returning on the beach, you can follow a trail that heads up the bluff and return to the horseshoe-shaped pond you passed earlier.

HOAX AND HISTORY: WHERE DID DRAKE LAND?

A long-standing controversy surrounds the story of Francis Drake's visit to the California coast. Drake's own log of his voyage has not resurfaced since he presented it to Queen Elizabeth I upon his return to England, so most of what we know about Drake comes from second-hand accounts of the journal of his chaplain, Francis Fletcher; Fletcher's original log, however, has also apparently been lost. Two books, written in 1589 and 1628, which relied on Fletcher's journal, are among the few sources of information we have today about Drake's landing.

We do know that in 1579, Francis Drake sailed the California coast, looking for a sheltered harbor to careen his ship, the *Golden Hinde*, and to prepare it for the long voyage home. Having pillaged vast treasures from Spanish settlements in South America, Drake had decided it best to return to England across the Pacific. According to Fletcher's journal, on June 17, Drake found a suitable harbor in a place where "nipping colds and stinking fogges" obscured the sun and stars for two weeks. The exact location of this harbor is the source of the controversy. The description of the site—which he called Nova Albion because the white banks and cliffs reminded him of home—and of the welcoming Native

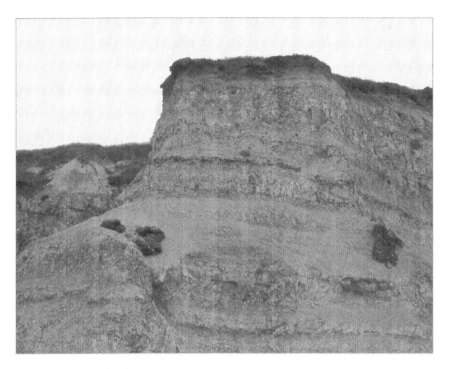

Eroding cliffs at Drakes Beach

Americans who greeted the crew with gifts, leads most historians to agree that it was present-day Drakes Bay; but others argue that the northwest shore of San Francisco Bay, Bolinas Lagoon, and Bodega and Tomales bays are all possibilities. One historian even contends that he may have landed in Coos Bay, Oregon! A map depicting the site, published by a Flemish cartographer in 1589, is sufficiently vague as to fit any of these spots.

A plate of brass inscribed with Drake's words was discovered in 1936 and further fanned the flames of controversy. Originally considered genuine, the plate was placed on display in The Bancroft Library at the University of California, Berkeley. Metallurgical tests later called its authenticity into question, and in 2003 the plate was confirmed to be a hoax, part of an elaborate and playful scheme dreamed up by local historians.

Although Drake's precise landing site remains a mystery, most historians are convinced that the bay that today bears his name was indeed where Drake and the *Golden Hinde* reposed in 1579. A large granite cross at the north edge of the Drakes Beach parking lot—west of the entrance road—and a bronze plaque at the south edge of the lot commemorate Drake.

►POINT REYES BEACH (NORTH AND SOUTH)

You can't beat this 11-mile stretch of sand for a long beach walk. Bring the dog and spend a few hours walking and building driftwood sculptures.

Driving Directions: You can reach Point Reyes Beach, also called the Great Beach, via two entrances, north and south. From the Bear Valley Visitor Center, return to Bear Valley Road and turn left. In 2 miles, turn left again on Sir Francis Drake Highway and continue through Inverness to the junction with Pierce Point Road (2.5 miles past Inverness). Bear left to stay on Sir Francis Drake and after 5.5 miles, turn right to on the road to North Beach. Continue 2.5 miles beyond on Sir Francis Drake to reach the turnoff to South Beach.

Facilities: Water, restrooms, picnic tables

Regulations: Dogs allowed on a 6-foot maximum leash; dog restrictions during snowy plover nesting season; no swimming or wading due to dangerous surf

The Beach: As you approach Point Reyes Beach, the grasslands of the outer point slope toward the coast and the hills roll into sandy dunes. Only sparsely covered by vegetation, the dunes often reach far inland, blown across the grasslands by the wind. The Great Beach itself stretches for 11 miles along the Pacific Coast, exposed to high winds from the northwest and crashing surf with a strong undertow. The long and wild strand is perfect for an exhilarating walk, run, or romp with the dog, but the cold and rough water is not the place for a swim. Abundant driftwood in fantastic shapes gathers on this beach, making good material for sculptures. In winter and spring, you might spot migrating whales.

If you visit when the beach is enveloped in fog or battered by strong winds, it won't be hard to imagine the shipwrecks that beset these shores, even after the light-

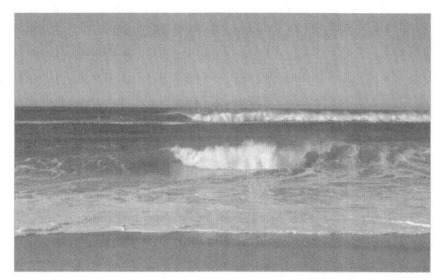

Surf at Point Reyes Beach

house was built in 1870. A Coast Guard lifesaving station operated on the beach from 1890 until 1927, but the winds and weather proved too much even for the rescue station, and it was moved to more sheltered Drakes Bay. A display at the lighthouse relates several colorful stories about shipwrecks at Point Reyes and you can visit the historic Lifeboat Station at Chimney Rock (see page 159).

▶ CHIMNEY ROCK TRAILHEAD

Chimney Rock is at its peak in spring, when wildflowers coat the grasslands and whales skirt the point on their migratory journey north, but all times of year warrant a visit. Sea lions and porpoises frolic in the waters, and cormorants and other pelagic birds frequent the cliffs and offshore rocks. In winter, a colony of elephant seals takes over a cove along Drakes Bay, which you can view from an overlook just a short walk from the Chimney Rock parking area. Come prepared for wind and fog: other than the lighthouse, probably no place is as blustery as Chimney Rock on a spring day.

Facilities: Toilets, wind shelter at the trailhead
Regulations: No bikes, horses, or dogs
Driving Directions: From the Bear Valley Visitor Center, return to Bear Valley Road and turn left. In 2 miles, turn left again on Sir Francis Drake Highway and continue through Inverness to the junction with Pierce Point Road (2.5 miles past Inverness). Bear left to stay on Sir Francis Drake, and 11.5 miles past the junction turn left on a narrow road, signed to CHIMNEY ROCK. Continue 1 mile to the parking lot.

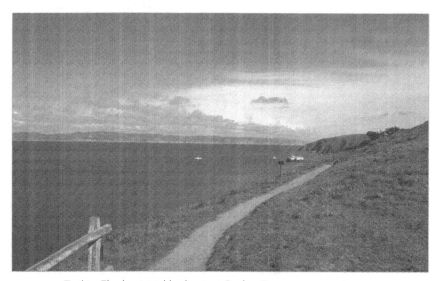

Trail to Elephant seal lookout on Drakes Bay

Note: On weekends and holidays from late December through mid-April, Sir Francis Drake Highway is closed at South Beach. A shuttle-bus service leaves from the Drakes Beach parking lot and takes visitors to the lighthouse and Chimney Rock. Reservations are not required. Adult tickets cost $4; children 12 and under ride free. See page 96 for more information.

Elephant Seal Overlook
Distance: 0.6 mile round trip

On weekends and holidays between late November and early March, trained docents set up spotting scopes and answer your questions at the Elephant Seal Overlook.

From the parking lot, signs direct you to a short dirt trail that branches left from the paved road. After 0.3 mile along the bluff, you reach an overlook with

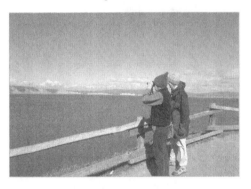

Looking for elephant seals

a great view of an elephant seal colony in a protected cove on Drakes Bay. With the aid of the scopes or binoculars, you can get an up-close view of the seals and watch birthings and male dominance contests. You might hear the male's loud calls as well.

Males usually arrive at Point Reyes by late November and begin to establish dominance, producing loud, drum-like noises and inflating their huge (elephant-like) noses. Pregnant females come shortly thereafter and give birth to their pups within a week of arrival. Juveniles and subadults also gather, pushing the number of animals in the colony to near 200.

These enormous mammals may look like sluggish lumps on land, but don't let their appearance fool you: elephant seals migrate over 14,000 miles on two yearly journeys and dive to depths of over 2000 feet on average (the deepest recorded dive is over 5800 feet). Extraordinary animals, elephant seals are perfectly adapted to their environment: they store oxygen in their blood rather than in their lungs, allowing them to stay underwater far longer than most mammals. They use their large eyes to locate food in the deep waters that are their feeding grounds.

In 1981, an elephant seal pup was born at Point Reyes for the first time in the 20th century, and in recent years they have become a common sight on beaches here. Northern elephant seals were once abundant along the Pacific Coast from Baja California to Point Reyes, but were hunted to near extinction in the 1800s, when probably only a few hundred seals remained. In the 1900s, the seals slowly regained prominence along the coast and today, their population is estimated to be over 150,000.

Lifeboat Station

Point Reyes is notorious for the shipwrecks that repeatedly landed on the peninsula's rocky promontories and beaches. Even after the lighthouse was built in 1870 to warn ships of the point, the wrecks continued. In 1888, the Coast Guard built a lifesaving station on South Beach. After nearly four decades on the storm-ridden Pacific beach, the Coast Guard moved operations to the sheltered waters of Drakes Bay at Chimney Rock. This station functioned until 1968, when the Coast Guard abandoned it for a newer facility in Bodega Bay. The National Park Service restored the station, and in 1990 it was declared a National Historic Landmark.

Hours: Open weekends and holidays from late December to April, 12 P.M. to 4 P.M.; closed December 25.

Chimney Rock Trail

Trip 20

Distance: 1.8 miles
Type: Out-and-back
Difficulty: Easy

A narrow path from the parking lot heads toward the coastal promontory. The lifeboat station is below you, overlooking the waters of Drakes Bay. Spring often brings windy and sunny days, with stunning contrasts between billowing white clouds against blue sky and stark white cliffs behind sparkling aquamarine waters. Long grasses dance in the wind, revealing splashes of color on green hillsides.

Flowers begin appearing by early March, and you might think the 20 or so early season species you see are impressive, but nothing prepares you for the show just a few weeks later, when the vivid green slopes of the promontory dance with color. Botanists have documented 80 different flower species on Chimney Rock.

After about a half mile on the trail, you'll see evidence of severe landslides above the Pacific Coast, where slopes have buckled and slid to rocky, wave-beaten coves. After a short rise, the main trail continues straight and several small trails branch to the right. If you take these trails, proceed with extreme caution. You will be above the landslides you witnessed from below and will see that where many a previous trail went, the land has since given way. The use trails converge on a plateau high above the turbulent Pacific waters and follow the western slope of the point to its tip.

The main trail continues roughly down the middle of the point, passing a left-branching side trail that detours above the more sheltered waters of Drakes

Bay and rejoins the main trail near the tip. From the vantage point at the tip of Chimney Rock, on clear days you'll have spectacular southward views that stretch beyond the Marin Headlands and San Francisco to San Pedro Point near Half Moon Bay. Look for porpoises and seals frolicking just offshore, and for whales on their annual migration in January, March, and April.

Algae Art

Steep cliffs drop from the grassy promontory of Chimney Rock to small rocky coves along Drakes Bay. Arresting orange splotches cover the cliffs, contrasting with the deep blue of the bay and the springtime green of the hills. The organism responsible for these colorful works of modern art is algae. Marine algae come in three types—green, brown, and red—and their name does not necessarily correspond to the color we see. The orange on the cliffs is actually a green alga colored by a red pigment in its chlorophyll.

►THE LIGHTHOUSE

At the very tip of Point Reyes itself, the historic Point Reyes lighthouse still casts its warning beam out to sea. The lighthouse is an ideal vantage point from which to scan the Pacific for whales. While you're there, visit the Sea Lion Overlook and learn about lighthouse history at the visitor center.

Driving Directions: From the Bear Valley Visitor Center, return to Bear Valley Road and turn left. In 2 miles, turn left again on Sir Francis Drake Highway and continue through Inverness to the junction with Pierce Point Road (2.5 miles past Inverness). Bear left to stay on Sir Francis Drake and continue to the lighthouse parking area (about 45 minutes from Bear Valley). The Lighthouse Visitor Center is about half a mile up a paved road from the parking area. Some disabled parking is available closer to the visitor center.

Note: On weekends and holidays from late December through mid-April, Sir Francis Drake Highway is closed at South Beach. A shuttle-bus service leaves from the Drakes Beach parking lot and takes visitors to the lighthouse and Chimney Rock. Reservations are not required. Adult tickets cost $4; children 12 and under ride free. See page 96 for more information.

Hours: Stair access to lighthouse open Thursday through Monday, 10 A.M. to 4:30 P.M.; Lens Room open Thursday through Monday, 2:30 P.M. to 4 P.M.; both are closed when winds exceed 40 miles per hour, in heavy fog, and on December 25.

Facilities: Restrooms and water at the visitor center; wheelchair-accessible

Regulations: No bikes, horses, or dogs

Description: From the parking lot, walk about a half mile up the paved road to the visitor center. Cypress trees grace the bluffs along the way, and you have fantastic views of the Great Beach sweeping north to meet the rocky cliffs of

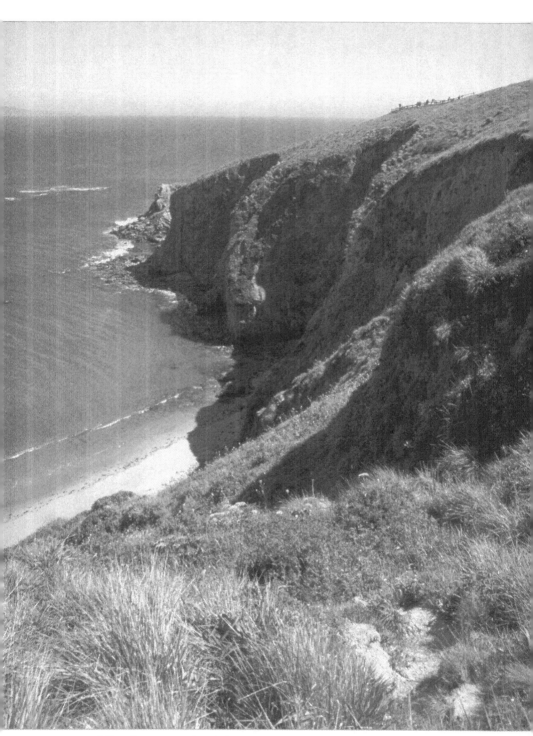

Cliffs with orange-colored algae at Chimney Rock

Tomales Point. Succulents and wildflowers adorn the cliffs, and interpretive plaques inform you about the Cordell Bank National Marine Sanctuary and the intriguing life of the lichens that also grow on the cliffs. You pass park residences and reach the visitor center (see below).

The historic lighthouse itself is some 300 steps down the cliff, perched just 240 feet above the crashing Pacific. It is well worth the walk, but if you don't want to face the climb back up—equivalent to a 30-story building—you can look for whales and enjoy the view from the viewing spot at the top of the stairs.

Visitor Center
Phone: (415) 669-1534
Hours: 10 A.M. to 4:30 P.M., Thursday through Monday; closed December 25
Facilities: Restrooms and water; wheelchair-accessible
At the visitor center you can see historic photographs of shipwrecks and lighthouse keepers, learn about local birds, and touch whale baleen. A small bookstore sells maps, books, and educational materials.

On weekend afternoons April through December, "A Look Into the Lens" presents the history of the lighthouse. On the first and third Saturday of each month, April through December, you can see the lighthouse light illuminated. Call (415) 669-1534 for details and to make reservations.

Whale-watching at the Lighthouse
The lighthouse is one of the best spots in Point Reyes to view whales. The southern migration of gray whales, from their feeding grounds in Alaska to mating and breeding sites in Baja, peaks in January; in late March and early April gray whales return north, babies in tow, and they often travel closer to shore. An overlook above the lighthouse provides a viewing platform for whale-watchers who don't want to descend the 300 steps.

To find out in advance about weather conditions and whale activity, call the Bear Valley or Lighthouse visitor centers. For more information about whales and whale-watching at Point Reyes, see page73–75.

Sea Lion Overlook
A great place to look for sea lions, whales, and seabirds, this cliff-side viewing point is just below the lighthouse parking lot. Descend 54 steps to search the rocky shoreline for sea lions. You may hear them long before you see them, as sea lions are known for their loud barking. Although sea lions are often confused with harbor seals, several distinct features distinguish the two species: sea lions have external ear flaps, unlike harbor seals. Because they can rotate their pelvis, sea lions can walk easily using their back flippers, whereas harbor seals scoot along on their bellies. You might also see whales and Brandt's cormorants from this vantage point.

After numerous ships met their end on the rocky points and beaches along this coast, the Point Reyes lighthouse was built in 1870. The lighthouse's location halfway down the 600-foot cliff was not an arbitrary one. At the recently built Point Bonita lighthouse, atop a cliff in the Marin Headlands, the high light was often obscured by fog. Although the location of the Point Reyes lighthouse increased the expense and the difficulty of constructing and provisioning the lighthouse, it resulted in a more useful warning station. The original light contained an intricate Fresnel lens imported from France. Using only light from four oil-burning wicks, it could be seen as far as 24 nautical miles out to sea.

As you might imagine, the isolated life of the lighthouse keeper was not an easy one. Wretched weather, hard work, and the din of the foghorn conspired against keepers; as one log entry reveals, in 1889 an assistant "went crazy and was handed over to the constable in Olema."

Despite the prime location, a strong light, and a foghorn, the lighthouse was unable to prevail over the fog, and did not put a stop to shipwrecks off the coast of Point Reyes. Point Reyes is the foggiest place on the Pacific Coast, and is second only to Nantucket Island in all of North America; visibility can be as little as 10 feet in heavy fogs. Coastal topography added to the problem: the Point Reyes headlands, extending 10 miles into the ocean, often surprised ships entering or leaving San Francisco Bay.

The lighthouse is still in operation today, although a new computer-operated light has replaced the old one. Visit the lighthouse to learn about its fascinating history firsthand. In the lens room (when staffed), you can see the original clockworks and Fresnel lens, more than 130 years old but still in working condition.

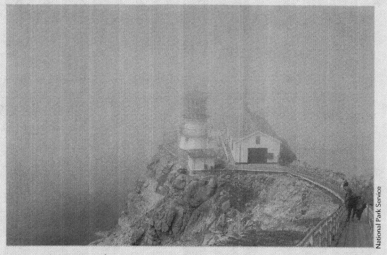

National Park Service

Lighthouse in fog

PIERCE POINT ROAD TRAILS AND BEACHES

Pierce Point Road crosses the sweeping moors of the northern end of Point Reyes. From bishop-pine–studded Inverness Ridge, rolling pastureland extends to the Pacific Ocean, splashed with brilliant yellow flowers in spring. Some days, thick masses of fog, much-bemoaned by early visitors and ranchers, hangs heavy over this long spit, enveloping you in an enchanting misty world. Other days, the fog billows in fits and starts, blowing across the headlands and dipping into low valleys, then lifting to reveal the rocky Pacific coast and the gentle bayside.

This is dairy country, and you'll pass several working historic ranches. Cows graze the hillsides and lend a pungent smell to the breeze. Trailheads along the road offer short walks to beaches on the Pacific Coast and Tomales Bay. You'll find long shoreline strolls, and a hike to the northernmost tip of the peninsula. Plan on a 35- to 40-minute drive from Bear Valley to Pierce Point Ranch.

For trails in Tomales Bay State Park, see pages 207–214.

Trip 21 Marshall Beach and Lairds Landing trails

You'll find a serene beach at the end of this short route and fantastic views and great spring wildflowers along the way. Enjoyable for all, the wide trail makes it especially good for bikes.

Distance: 2.4 miles round trip
Type: Out-and-back
Difficulty: Easy
Facilities: Toilets, trash cans at beach
Regulations: No dogs, no fires, no motor vehicles; camping by permit only
Driving Directions: From the Bear Valley Visitor Center, turn left on Bear Valley Road; veer left on Sir Francis Drake Highway, and continue through Inverness. Veer right on Pierce Point Road (2.5 miles beyond Inverness). After a little over a mile, just past Tomales Bay State Park, turn right on Duck Cove/Marshall Beach Road, signed L RANCH. After 2.5 miles on a smooth dirt road, you reach a dirt parking area. (Bikes can start at the junction of Pierce Point and Duck Cove/Marshall Beach roads for a 7.5-mile round-trip ride to the beach.)

At the northern edge of the parking area, your trail is marked to Marshall Beach; another trail leads to Lairds Landing, an adjacent cove along the bay. Fairly level at first, the trail affords exceptional views to the east and west, where grasslands descend to the blue waters of the Pacific Ocean and of Tomales Bay. In spring, wildflowers color the green hillsides, large clusters of iris sprout beneath coyote bush, and blue-eyed grass, sun cups, buttercups, beach strawberry, and poppies grow along the trail.

You soon pass through two cattle stiles and begin to descend toward the narrow bay. Views south stretch to Black Mountain, Mt. Wittenberg, Point Reyes Hill, and Mt. Vision; to the north, you can see Hog Island and Dillon Beach; directly across the bay, the white Victorian buildings of the Audubon Canyon Ranch Cypress Grove Preserve perch on the shore. The rounded curves of windswept trees cascade down the hillside to the bay, which glistens beneath sunny skies. Look for the fuzzy lavender petals of pussy ears (*Calochortus tolmiei*) in spring as you pass a grassy sward on your left.

As you near the beach, coyote bush, coffeeberry, honeysuckle, and poison oak grow densely along the trail, intertwined with sprawling strands of wild cucumber. Moss hangs from Monterey cypress branches, evidence of the fog that often sweeps across these hillsides. Beneath the shade of cypress you arrive at the broad, curved beach. Lairds Landing is the eucalyptus-cloaked cove to the south, reachable from Marshall Beach at low tide. A path leads north over a low grassy bluff to another sandy cove. At the far end of this cove, you can climb over the barnacled rocks and peek around the cliff to catch sight of the mouth of Tomales Bay.

The beach was named for Robert Marshall, a rancher who bought this property in 1960—no relation to the Marshall brothers who founded the town across Tomales Bay.

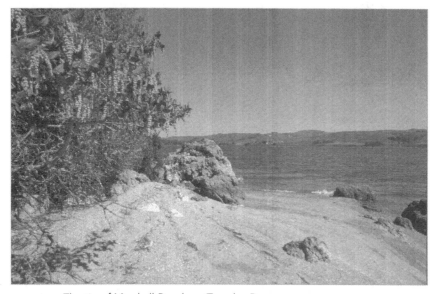

The tip of Marshall Beach on Tomales Bay

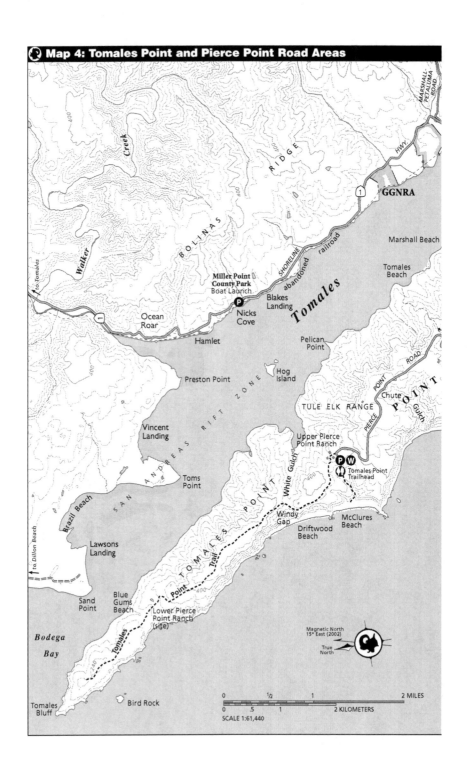

Map 4: Tomales Point and Pierce Point Road Areas

GGNRA

Marshall Beach

Tomales Beach

Miller Point
County Park
Boat Launch

Blakes Landing

Nicks Cove

Ocean Roar

Hamlet

Pelican Point

Preston Point

Hog Island

TULE ELK RANGE

Chute Gulch

Vincent Landing

Upper Pierce Point Ranch

Tomales Point Trailhead

Toms Point

White Gulch

McClures Beach

Brazil Beach

Windy Gap

Driftwood Beach

Lawsons Landing

Sand Point

Blue Gums Beach

Lower Pierce Point Ranch (site)

Bodega Bay

Magnetic North
15° East (2002)

True North

Tomales Bluff

Bird Rock

0   ½   1   2 MILES

0   .5   1   2 KILOMETERS

SCALE 1:61,440

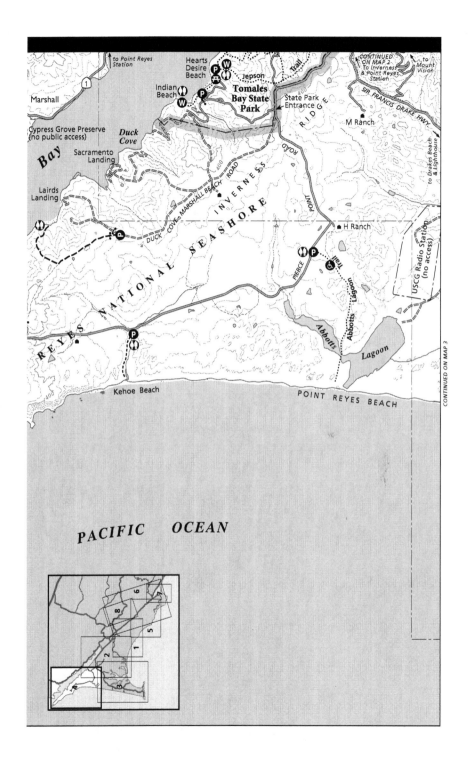

to Point Reyes
Station

Hearts
Desire
Beach

Jepson

Trail

CONTINUED
ON MAP 2
To Inverness
& Point Reyes
Station

to
Mount
Vision

Marshall

Indian
Beach

**Tomales
Bay State
Park**

State Park
Entrance

M Ranch

SIR FRANCIS DRAKE HWY.

Cypress Grove Preserve
(no public access)

*Duck
Cove*

Bay

Sacramento
Landing

RIDGE

to Drakes Beach
& Lighthouse

Lairds
Landing

INVERNESS

DUCK COVE—MARSHALL BEACH ROAD

ROAD

400

H Ranch

USCG Radio Station
(no access)

REYES NATIONAL SEASHORE

PIERCE POINT

Trail

Abbotts Lagoon

CONTINUED ON MAP 3

Abbotts

Lagoon

400

Kehoe Beach

POINT REYES BEACH

PACIFIC OCEAN

6

8

5

2

1

3

Abbotts Lagoon Trail

A freshwater marsh, brackish lagoon, and open ocean all provide prime birdwatching and wildflower viewing on this easy ramble.

> **Distance:** 2.2 miles round trip to lagoon; 3.2 miles round trip to beach
> **Type:** Out-and-back
> **Difficulty:** Easy
> **Facilities:** Toilets; no water; first 0.4-mile wheelchair-accessible
> **Regulations:** No dogs
> **Driving Directions:** From the Bear Valley Visitor Center, turn left on Bear Valley Road; veer left on Sir Francis Drake Highway, and continue through Inverness. Veer right on Pierce Point Road (2.5 miles beyond Inverness) and follow it 3.4 miles to the trailhead on the left.

From the trailhead, Abbotts Lagoon's two freshwater ponds appear as a blue splash of color in the surrounding pastureland. These two ponds are just a small part of the 282-acre lagoon. Tucked behind a knoll and connected to the ponds by a spillway, a large, brackish lagoon borders the beach.

The initial half-mile of trail, level and well-graded, is wheelchair-accessible. Grasses, coyote bush, ferns, and blackberry border the trail, and in spring, poppies, light blue iris, and bright yellow fiddleneck brighten the surrounding green fields. As the trail nears the ponds, salmonberry and blackberry amass in large clusters, and wild cucumber runs rampant over the coastal scrub bushes. Tules

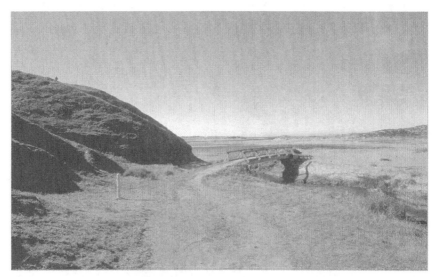

Bridge at Abbotts Lagoon between freshwater and brackish lagoons

and reeds grow in moist swales. A couple of wooden benches invite you to rest and informative plaques reveal facts about the lagoon's birdlife.

A small bridge crosses the natural spillway between the freshwater ponds and the brackish lagoon (1.1 miles) and leads onto a broad dune that extends to the ocean. Skirt the lagoon, looking for shorebirds foraging along the water's edge. Caspian terns, coots, western and pied-billed grebes are among those you may see feasting on clams, snails, crabs, and worms, and diving for small fish. A sandbar protects the lagoon from tidal influences, although severe winter storms can wash it away, letting the ocean waters in. The sand eventually builds up again and seals off the opening.

To find out why Abbotts Lagoon is known as a prime wildflower-viewing spot, take the path up the low hillside just before crossing the bridge at 1.1 miles. In spring, goldfields (*Lasthenia crysotoma*) coat the slope along the narrow path, and the grassy mesa-top shimmers with iris (*Iris douglasii*), pussy ears (*Calochortus tolmeii*), buttercups (*Ranunculus californicus*), and blue-eyed grass (*Sisyrinchium bellum*). Vistas across the lagoon take in the coast and the lighthouse point in the south; look north across the smooth, windswept dune to the muted greens of grassy hillsides and cows grazing the pastures beyond.

Ground-hugging plants grow in small stands on the dunes, including Tidestrom's lupine (*Lupinus tidestromii*), beach layia (*Layia carnosa*), and beach strawberry (*Fragaria chiloensis*). Invasive European beachgrass and ice plant have taken over much of the dunes and threaten the survival of many of the native plants and animals. (See page 31 about the dune restoration project at Abbotts Lagoon.)

Beyond the dunes, a glorious strip of smooth beach (Point Reyes Beach) stretches for miles in both directions. You can follow the coastline north toward Kehoe Beach, with the craggy cliffs of Tomales Point in the distance, or south along the extensive beach that culminates at the lighthouse point.

▶ KEHOE BEACH

A short path leads to Kehoe Beach, where 10 miles of uninterrupted, smooth sand stretch southward. Tidepools, marsh birds, and spectacular wildflowers make Kehoe a great place to spend an afternoon, and it is one of the few beaches in the seashore that allow dogs.

Distance: 0.6 mile-path to the beach
Facilities: Toilet by roadside parking
Regulations: Dogs on maximum 6-foot leash
Driving Directions: From the Bear Valley Visitor Center, turn left on Bear Valley Road; veer left on Sir Francis Drake Highway, and continue through Inverness. Veer right on Pierce Point Road (2.5 miles beyond Inverness) and follow it for 5.5 miles to the roadside parking at a sign for Kehoe Beach.

At first glance, the wild, uninhabited dunes around Abbotts Lagoon would seem an ideal environment for western snowy plovers (*Charadrius alexandrinus*). These small, 16 centimeter-tall shorebirds are identified by their thin black bill, a distinct black patch behind the eye, and an incomplete necklace of black extending on either side of the throat. The rotund plovers nest on sandy beaches and around lagoons and feed on invertebrates. But the snowy plover population at Abbotts Lagoon and other nesting areas in Point Reyes and elsewhere has declined over the past 30 years, and plovers are now considered a federally threatened species.

Although protected from urbanization and development by national seashore status, Point Reyes beaches are not immune to habitat destruction, and even here, human activities can put a species at risk. Two nonnative plants—European dunegrass (*Ammophila arenaria*) and ice plant (*Mesembryanthemum*)—first planted on Point Reyes beaches to stabilize shifting dunes, have rapidly spread across the sand, forming thick mats that shut out other plant species and alter the dune habitat. Snowy plovers, who prefer a more open habitat, have moved their nests onto the beach, which has been narrowed by the growth of the nonnative dunegrass.

On the narrow, open beach, the birds are exposed to wind and storms, as well as to people, who unwittingly threaten plover populations. To make matters worse, plover breeding season, mid-March through September, coincides with human beach-going season. Even our most innocuous activities, like picnicking on the beach, increase the plovers' chance of predation. Our food scraps draw gulls, ravens, skunks, raccoons, foxes, and other opportunistic feeders to the beach; when we walk dogs or ride horses near plover nests, we cause adults to leave their nestside post, and the unprotected eggs and chicks become easy prey for the predators our picnic attracted. The driftwood sculptures we build in the sand provide perches for raptors waiting to prey on unattended nests.

In a joint project, the National Park Service and Point Reyes Bird Observatory are working to learn more about what activities harm plovers and to what extent. Monitors found that chick deaths increased 150 percent on weekends over weekdays. To protect plover nests, the park has roped off important breeding areas along Point Reyes Beach, including the sections by Abbotts Lagoon. Wire fencing with twine around the top, called exclosures, allow plovers to go in and out of nests but protect eggs and chicks from predators like ravens, raptors, and gulls. In addition, the park has closed about three miles of Point Reyes Beach to dogs during peak breeding season.

The Beach: A 0.6-mile trail leads from the road to the beach, following a small creek that becomes the freshwater Kehoe Marsh. Yellow bush lupine and tall grasses sprawl over the hillsides. Look for light blue phacelia flowers peeking above masses of fern-like leaves. Dune grasses whip in the wind, the sandy trail crests a small rise, and the white, sandy beach and the vast Pacific spread before you.

Just before you descend the dune to the beach, a small path heads up the bluffs and leads across stunning, wildflower-studded pastures overlooking the coast. In spring, tidy tips, baby blue eyes, iris, goldfields, poppies, and lupine coat the slopes. These cliffs offer a good vantage point to scan the water for whales in winter and early spring.

For good tidepooling opportunities, head north along the sand toward the rocky termination of the Great Beach. Geology buffs will take interest in the clearly visible fault that cuts through the cliffs at the north end of the beach. In the steep cliff walls, you can see the young marine rock called Lairds sandstone, which overlays the peninsula's granitic baserock. In spring, the cliffs glow with the bright yellow flowers of lizard tail.

Kehoe Beach to Abbotts Lagoon

Trip 23

Birdwatching, wildflower viewing, and beachwalking—this shuttle hike has it all. You follow a short path along a creek to freshwater Kehoe Marsh and the Great Beach beyond. After a couple of miles on the beach, you head across the sweeping dunes at Abbotts Lagoon. These freshwater and brackish ponds provide ample habitat for birds and the surrounding hillsides glow with wildflowers come spring.

Distance: 4.7 miles one-way
Type: Shuttle
Difficulty: Easy
Facilities: Toilet at Abbotts Lagoon and Kehoe parking areas; no water
Regulations: Dogs on maximum six-foot leash
Driving Directions: From the Bear Valley Visitor Center, turn left on Bear Valley Road; veer left on Sir Francis Drake Highway, and continue through Inverness. Veer right on Pierce Point Road (2.5 miles beyond Inverness) and follow it for 5.5 miles to the roadside parking at a sign for Kehoe Beach.

The sandy trail follows a small creek that runs to freshwater Kehoe Marsh, just behind the beach. In spring, light blue phacelia flowers mingle among yellow bush lupine beside the trail, and tall grasses sprawl over the hillsides. After about

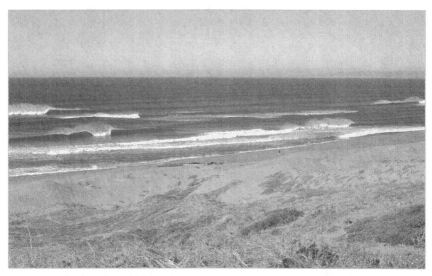

The beach at Abbotts Lagoon

a half mile, you crest a small rise among coarse dune grasses and arrive at a long strip of beach.

Head southward along the sand, taking in views of the lighthouse point at the distant tip of this 11-mile beach. After 2.5 miles on the sand, look for the low sandbar between the beach and the brackish lagoon beyond. Head inland across the dunes, staying on the left (north) side of the lagoon. In severe winter storms, the sandbar sometimes breeches and ocean water surges into the lagoon; sand eventually builds up again and seals off the lagoon. After about half a mile, you cross a wooden bridge between the lagoon and two upper ponds. Take the short path up the hillside on the right to see a dramatic display of spring wildflowers—goldfields, lupine, pussy ears, and blue-eyed grass. Return to the main trail along the fresh-water upper ponds to reach the Abbotts Lagoon parking area, 1.1 miles from the bridge.

Abbotts Lagoon is one of the best birding spots in the seashore, especially during the fall migration. The combination of ocean, brackish lagoon, and freshwater pond provides ample habitat for sea-, marsh-, and shorebirds and the raptors that prey on them.

► MCCLURES BEACH

The northernmost beach on the peninsula, rugged McClures Beach is as entrancing in a misty fog as it is in sparkling sun. Seabirds flock to the offshore granite rocks, beachside cliffs teem with wildflowers, and fascinating inverte-brates live in tidepools.

McClures was the second piece of land on the peninsula to become a public park. (Drakes Beach, pages 152–155 was the first). In 1942, Margaret McClure

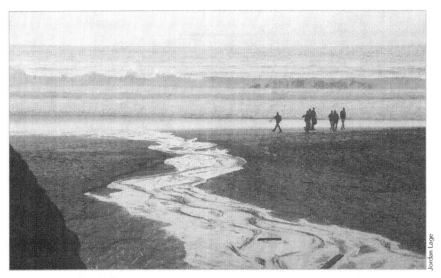

McClures Beach at sunset

turned over 2.9 acres of her Pierce Point property to the county; in return, they improved the access road to her ranch, eliminating long trips into town on a muddy and rutted road, and built a parking lot and public-access path to the beach. In 1965, the National Park Service incorporated the beach into the newly created national seashore.

Distance: 0.4-mile path to the beach
Facilities: Toilets in parking lot; water, phone at Pierce Point Ranch, 0.2 mile up the road
Regulations: No dogs; no swimming or wading
Driving Directions: From the Bear Valley Visitor Center, turn left on Bear Valley Road; veer left on Sir Francis Drake Highway, and continue through Inverness. Veer right on Pierce Point Road (2.5 miles beyond Inverness) and follow it to the end (about 35 to 40 minutes from the visitor center).
The Beach: A short, sandy trail descends next to a small creekbed to reach McClures Beach. The soil on the steep and eroded hillsides has given way to severe landslides over the years. In season, the trail is flush with brightly colored wild-flowers. Yellow and blue lupine, yellow-eyed grass, and wild radish bloom through-out the spring and into summer, and white flowers decorate the sprawling branches of morning glory. Sticky monkeyflower often blooms well into fall, when the fleshy leaves of ice plant turn bright magenta. In spring and fall, migrating birds frequent the streamside willows below the trail, seeking freshwater.

One of the best beaches at Point Reyes, McClures feels wild and remote. High granite cliffs enclose the beach, less than a mile in length. In the cliffs at the south-ern end of the sand, look for shiny outcroppings of metamorphic rocks, the oldest rocks on the Point Reyes peninsula. Water trickles down the eroding cliffs in wet months, and a rich and colorful array of plants grows on the rocky walls and in lush seeps: dudleya, iris, fiddleneck, monkeyflower, lizard tail, and gumplant.

At low tide, a defile in the rocks that enclose the beach to the south leads to an adjacent narrow spit of sand. Just offshore, the sea stack called Elephant Rocks was once part of the cliff; ocean waves have worn away the connecting rocks, and these harder pillars remain. Look for cormorants on the rocks.

To the north, rugged cliffs extend beyond the beach and along the length of Tomales Point above small, rocky coves. McClures Beach is a good spot to explore tidepools.

Tomales Point Trail

The Tomales Point Trail, one of the most dramatic trips in the seashore, leads across an outlying spit of land to reach the northern-most spot on the peninsula. Tule elk roam the point, spring wildflow-ers bloom abundantly, and in the migratory seasons (fall and spring) red-tailed and kestrel hawks soar overhead and harrier hawks skim the contours of the land. The fairly level route along a former ranch road affords views east and west, to the Pacific Ocean and Tomales Bay. A self-guided tour of the historic ranch at the trailhead describes life on a Point Reyes dairy ranch and tells about the peninsula's famous but-ter industry. Come prepared for a chilly adventure, as these outer reaches of the point are often foggy and blustery.

Distance: 9.4 miles round trip to the tip
Type: Out-and-back
Difficulty: Moderate to strenuous
Facilities: Toilets at McClures Beach parking lot; no water
Regulations: Horses allowed; no bikes or dogs
Driving Directions: From the Bear Valley Visitor Center, turn left on Bear Valley Road; veer left on Sir Francis Drake Highway, and con-tinue through Inverness. Veer right on Pierce Point Road (2.5 miles beyond Inverness) and follow it to the end (about 35 to 40 minutes from the visitor center).

The hike begins just west of the ranch near a solitary stand of cypresses, a cou-ple of which have been uprooted in winter storms. The wide, sandy trail mean-ders through coyote bush, low-growing blue lupine, and the sweet-smelling yel-low flowers of coastal bush lupine (*Lupinus arboreus*). Wild radishes and California poppies also bloom in season. As you reach a high point just beyond the ranch, you can see Elephant Rock at the southern tip of McClures Beach.

The trail rounds a small knoll, and on clear days you have your first views of the Tomales Point peninsula as it stretches north, flanked by bay and ocean. Rocky outcrops dot the rounded hills, verdant in winter and spring. You gradually descend into appropriately named Windy Gap.

From Windy Gap you can see White Gulch, the inlet of Tomales Bay where Pierce Point butter was loaded onto schooners to be shipped to San Francisco. Look through the gulch to see Hog Island in the bay just beyond, reportedly named when a barge lost a load of pigs on its beach.

On a gentle ascent, you pass granitic outcroppings, good spots for a picnic or snack, and soon reach a level stretch high on the promontory. You can see east across Tomales Bay to the grassy hummocks beyond, and west to rocky and unreachable Pacific beaches below steep cliffs. The trail descends gradually to a stand of cypress and a small pond, the only remains of Lower Pierce Point Ranch, 3 miles from the trailhead. As it climbs the next hill, the trail narrows to a sandy path, flanked by fragrant lupine.

Less than a mile beyond the ranch site, you reach a bluff adjacent to Bird Rock, an offshore sea stack frequented by cormorants and pelicans. Beyond, the path peters out as it crosses sandy dunes, but you'll easily find your way through low stands of coyote bush, lupine, and morning glory. At 0.7 mile past Bird Rock, you reach the tip of Tomales Point, where a rocky granitic promontory teeters 30 feet above the ocean. Be careful on these precipitous and eroding cliffs overlooking the blustery gateway to Tomales Bay.

Development Visions for Tomales Bay

On clear days, or when the fog lifts intermittently, you can look east across Tomales Bay to cars speeding along Highway 1, the homes at Dillon Beach, and the campground at Lawson's Landing. The scale of this development is minor compared to the projected urbanization of the east shore of Tomales Bay in the 1960s—housing tracts, shopping malls, schools, and a junior college, linked by parkways and a major "scenic" highway between West Marin and the urban interior. An aqueduct was planned to bring water from the Russian River, and treated sewage would go directly into Tomales Bay.

▶ UPPER PIERCE POINT RANCH

The Tomales Point Trail begins at Upper Pierce Point Ranch, once the most prosperous dairy ranch at Point Reyes. In 1858, Solomon Pierce bought 2200 acres on the point from the Shafter brothers, who owned most of Point Reyes at that time, and established two dairies at Upper and Lower Pierce Point ranches. Celebrated for its soft yellow color and sweet taste, Pierce butter soon surpassed the Shafters' in quality and quantity. In the early days of the industry, schooners picked up butter from landings on Tomales Bay and delivered it to San

Francisco. After the North Pacific Coast Railroad line extended up the east side of Tomales Bay in 1875, butter was sent across the bay to the train and taken to Sausalito, where it completed the trip to San Francisco via ferry.

A small town grew up alongside the isolated ranches at Pierce Point, with a blacksmith shop, a carpenter shop (to make the butter boxes), barns, a schoolhouse, a laundry, and a well-stocked warehouse. In 1929, James McClure bought the ranch, and soon gave up butter-making to raise hogs and beef cattle. The National Park Service took over the ranch in 1973 and restored the original buildings. The ranch today provides an intriguing look into the dairying history of Point Reyes.

THE RETURN OF THE TULE ELK

After a 100-year hiatus, tule elk once again roam the coastal grasslands of Point Reyes. As you approach Pierce Point Ranch and walk the Tomales Point Trail, you're likely to see their large, graceful antlers and peculiar-shaped bodies. Large herds of tule elk populated Point Reyes for thousands of years, but hunting and a habitat shift from perennial bunchgrasses to European annuals proved a devastating combination for the elk.

In the mid-1800s, after tule elk were considered extinct throughout California, a Central Valley landowner discovered a small population on his land and protected them from disappearing completely. Tule elk gained official protection in 1971, and seven years later, the National Park Service reintroduced 10 elk to Tomales Point.

The Tomales Point population grew slowly at first, but by 2000 more than 400 inhabited 2,600 acres on the point, constricted by the natural boundaries of the bay and ocean on all but the southern edge, where a fence keeps them out of adjacent cattle-grazing land. Whereas some species at Point Reyes—like the snowy plover—struggle for survival, the thriving tule elk population has outgrown the contained reserve. The intense pressure on the land threatens rare plants and butterflies, and with so large a population, disease is more likely and forage is less available.

The Park Service has relocated about 30 elk to the wilderness area near Limantour. In another effort to reduce the growing population, the Park Service started a tule elk birth-control program. The immunocontraception works as a vaccine, and each year at the beginning of mating season female elk receive a

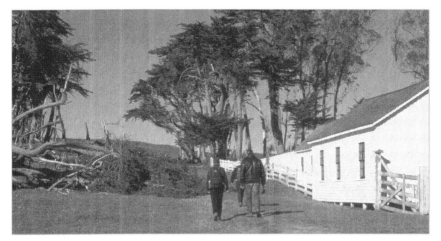

Historic dairy buildings at Upper Pierce Point Ranch

booster, injected with a dart rifle. The program has been successful so far, the last data reporting that the Tomales Point herd had leveled off at about 450 elk.

Elk-watching Tips

Tule elk rutting season lasts from mid-summer to mid-fall. Listen for the bugling sounds that male elk make to beckon females, but follow these guidelines, for your safety and for the health of the animals:

- Don't get too close to or come between tule elk—rutting bulls can be aggressive. If an elk begins to move away or looks nervous, you're too close. It's best to observe the elk with binoculars.
- Do not feed tule elk or any other wildlife.
- If you are observing the elk from your car, pull off the road completely.
- Don't startle the animals with loud speech or rapid movements.
- Don't feed the elk (or any other animals in the park) for their own health and for your safety.
- No pets or bikes allowed in tule elk areas.
- Do not collect or remove antlers; they are a calcium source for other wildlife like deer and rodents.

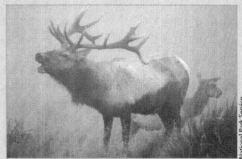

Bugling elk

FIVE BROOKS TRAILS AND BEACHES

Naturalists, hikers, and equestrians have plenty of options at the Five Brooks Trailhead. As you'll see from a glance at the map, this area, like much of Point Reyes, offers numerous route combinations, depending on the length, difficulty, and terrain you desire.

You can climb the forested eastern slope of Inverness Ridge and descend to the coast for a challenging full-day hike, or make a shorter loop with Firtop's peaceful meadow as your destination. The Rift Zone and Olema Valley trails offer easier walks along the San Andreas fault. Shuttle hikes to Bear Valley and Palomarin offer the possibility of an overnight at Wildcat Camp or Glen Camp along the way. The Stewart Trail from Five Brooks is the only bicycle route to Wildcat and Glen camps. Horses are allowed on all trails in the Five Brooks area, and nearby Stewart Horse Camp provides accommodations for equestrians.

At the mill pond near the trailhead, you'll find migratory landbirds in the willows and alders around the pond, especially between August and October. Turtles sometimes sun themselves on rocks in the pond, and in spring, hundreds of bullfrogs congregate to feast on tadpoles.

Logging in Point Reyes

The pond at Five Brooks, now habitat for birds, frogs, and turtles, was created to transport lumber from Inverness Ridge to a mill that stood nearby. In the 1950s, Marin County placed a tax on standing lumber, and many landowners sold their timber rights or started logging themselves. Sweet Lumber Company bought the rights to thousands of acres on Inverness Ridge and began logging the Douglas-firs, alarming local conservationists and proponents of the national seashore. The Park Service issued an emergency report, citing the danger of the proposed parkland being destroyed by logging. In 1962, the creation of the national seashore brought logging to an abrupt halt.

Driving Directions: From Olema, go south on Highway 1 for 3.5 miles to the signed Five Brooks Trailhead turnoff on the right side of the highway. From Bolinas Lagoon, go north on Highway 1 for 5 miles (from the northern end of the lagoon) and turn left at the sign. Follow the gravel road about one quarter of a mile to the trailhead.

Facilities: Water (by picnic area), toilets, picnic tables. Five Brooks Ranch offers guided rides, horse rentals, horse boarding, and hayrides. Open every day, 9 A.M. to 5 P.M. Reservations recommended. (415) 663-1570. www.fivebrooks.com.

Regulations: Bikes allowed on Stewart and Olema Valley trails and the Glen Camp Loop Trail as far as Glen Camp; horses allowed on all trails from Five Brooks; no dogs

Firtop via Greenpicker and Stewart trails

This route climbs the narrow, shaded Greenpicker Trail through a dense Douglas-fir forest. Rest or picnic at Firtop—an unexpected meadow ringed by trees—and return on the wide Stewart Trail, with views into pastoral Olema Valley and Bolinas Ridge beyond.

Distance: 6.4 miles
Type: Semi-loop
Difficulty: Moderate
Facilities: Toilets, water at Five Brooks Trailhead
Regulations: No dogs. Bikes allowed on Stewart Trail. Horses allowed on all trails.

Begin on the wide trail that skirts the mill pond, passing the Rift Zone Trail to arrive at a junction with the Stewart and Olema Valley trails, 0.1 mile from your car. Turn right on the Stewart Trail, an old ranch road. After an immediate and brief descent, you climb gently through a lush forest of Douglas-fir, bay laurel, big-leaf maple, hazelnut, and alder, with ferns and poison oak in the understory. The trail rings the deep ravine of a creek that descends the ridge to Olema Creek.

You leave the Stewart Trail 0.9 mile from the trailhead and pick up the narrow Greenpicker Trail, densely lined with vegetation. Although steeper than the Stewart Trail, Greenpicker is slightly shorter and provides a more varied route. Tanbark oak, bay laurel, and Douglas-fir trees overshadow masses of huckleberry bushes, and cow parsnip, blackberry, and sword fern crowd the edges of the path.

As you near Firtop, the trail widens and levels in a tunnel of Douglas-fir. The lush understory disappears, brown trunks stretch to towering heights, and dry needles cushion the trail. Continue straight at the first junction, on a wide, unsigned trail; the Greenpicker Trail goes right, to Glen Camp and coastal trails. In a short 0.1 mile, you reach Firtop.

At 1324 feet, Firtop crowns this southern branch of Inverness Ridge, although since its open patch of grass is surrounded by dense forest, it affords views neither of the coast nor of Olema Valley. Nevertheless, the peaceful retreat is ideal for a picnic or a nap in the sun.

From Firtop, return to the trailhead on the wide Stewart Trail, or extend this hike by continuing on one of the following trips to the coast or farther south along the ridge.

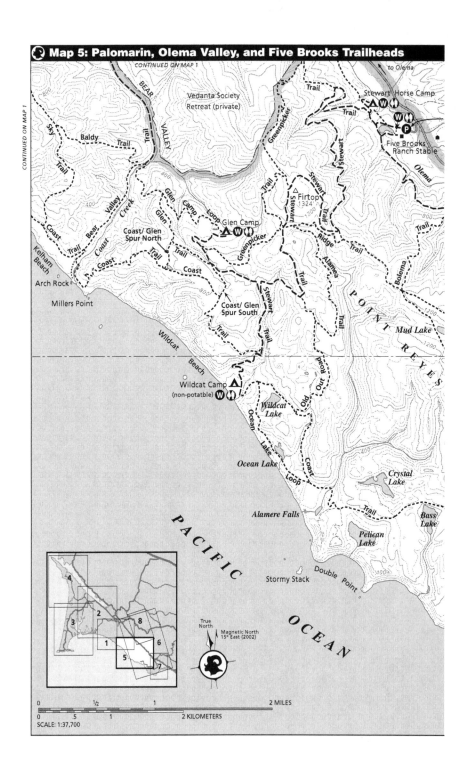

CONTINUED ON MAP 1

CONTINUED ON MAP 1

to Olema

Vedanta Society
Retreat (private)

Stewart Horse Camp

Five Brooks
Ranch Stable

Sky
Trail

Baldy

Trail

BEAR

VALLEY

Greenpicker

Trail

Stewart

Glen

Camp

Loop

Firtop
1324

Stewart

Stewart
Ridge
Trail

Valley

Creek

Bear

Coast

Glen

Glen Camp

Greenpicker

Alamea
Trail

Coast

Trail

Coast/ Glen
Spur North

Coast

Trail

Coast

Coast/ Glen
Spur South

Stewart

Bolema

Kelham
Beach

Arch Rock

POINT
REYES

Millers Point

Mud Lake

Wildcat
Beach

Old Out Road

Wildcat Camp
(non-potatble)

Wildcat
Lake

Ocean
Lake

Coast

Ocean Lake

Loop

Crystal
Lake

Trail

Alamere Falls

Bass
Lake

Pelican
Lake

PACIFIC

Stormy Stack

Double Point

O C E A N

4

2

8

3

1

6

5

7

True
North

Magnetic North
15° East (2002)

0   ½   1   2 MILES
0   .5   1   2 KILOMETERS
SCALE: 1:37,700

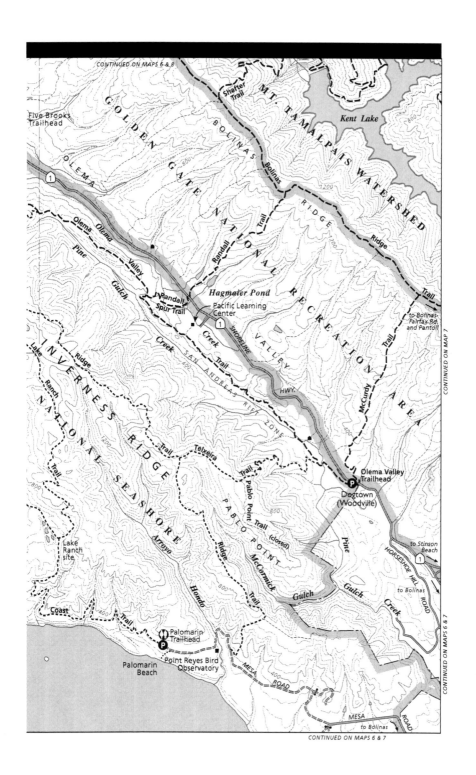

CONTINUED ON MAPS 6 & 8

MT. TAMALPAIS WATERSHED

Kent Lake

Shafter Trail

GOLDEN GATE NATIONAL RECREATION AREA

Five Brooks Trailhead

OLEMA

BOLINAS RIDGE

Bolinas

Ridge

Randall Trail

Trail

1

Olema

Olema Valley

Pine

Gulch

Randall Spur Trail

Hagmaier Pond

Pacific Learning Center

1

OLEMA VALLEY

Creek

Shoreline Trail

McCurdy

Trail

to Bolinas-Fairfax Rd. and Pantoll

CONTINUED ON MAP 7

INVERNESS RIDGE

Lake Ranch Trail

Creek Trail

SAN ANDREAS RIFT ZONE

HWY.

Ridge

Trail

Teixeira Trail

NATIONAL SEASHORE

Trail

PABLO POINT

Pablo Point Trail

Olema Valley Trailhead

P

Dogtown (Woodville)

to Stinson Beach

1

Lake Ranch site

Arroyo

Hondo

Ridge

Pablo Point Trail (closed)

McCormick Trail

Pine

Gulch

Gulch

HORSESHOE HILL

to Bolinas

Coast

Trail

Palomarin Trailhead

P

ROAD

CONTINUED ON MAPS 6 & 7

Palomarin Beach

Point Reyes Bird Observatory

MESA ROAD

MESA ROAD

to Bolinas

CONTINUED ON MAPS 6 & 7

Valley to Ridge Loop on Greenpicker, Ridge, Bolema, Olema Valley trails

A delightful romp through the woods, this route takes you up the ridge, circles Firtop, and then descends to the valley floor and returns along Olema Creek.

Distance: 7.1 miles
Type: Loop
Difficulty: Moderate to strenuous
Facilities: Toilets, water at Five Brooks Trailhead
Regulations: Horses allowed; no dogs, no bikes

The wide trail from the parking area skirts the mill pond and passes the Rift Zone Trail to arrive at a junction with the Stewart and Olema Valley trails, 0.1 mile from your car. Turn right on the Stewart Trail, an old ranch road, which makes an immediate and brief descent. You then climb gently through a lush forest of Douglas-fir, bay laurel, big-leaf maple, hazelnut, and alder, with ferns and poison oak in the understory. The trail rings the deep ravine of a creek that descends the ridge to Olema Creek.

You leave the Stewart Trail 0.9 mile from the trailhead and turn right on the narrow Greenpicker Trail. Lush vegetation lines the trail, shorter than the Stewart Trail although a bit steeper. Tanbark oak, bay laurel, and Douglas-fir trees overshadow masses of huckleberry bushes, and cow parsnip, blackberry, and sword ferns crowd the edges of the path.

You enter a dense corridor of Douglas-firs as you near Firtop, and the trail widens and levels. The lush understory disappears, brown trunks stretch to towering heights, and dry needles cushion the trail. At the first junction, go straight to make a 0.1-mile detour to Firtop. Otherwise, veer right to continue on the Greenpicker Trail, which wraps around the high knoll of Firtop and reaches another junction just 0.7 mile farther. Turn left to cross the Stewart Trail, now west of Firtop, and join the Ridge Trail, which begins in this clearing.

You may find the Ridge Trail muddy in spring, with elderberry and huckleberry bushes spilling onto its course. It is a delightful trail nevertheless, and worth enduring these small bothers. Sunlight wafts through the trees, splaying on the forest's varied palate of green. After half a mile, you veer right at a junction to continue on the Ridge Trail, now a wide track along the spine of the ridge, although still potentially muddy.

At the next intersection, 0.8 mile farther, turn left on the Bolema Trail, which runs steeply down the hillside. You may notice that the Douglas-fir forest on this southern part of Inverness Ridge is drier than that around Bear Valley, with fewer ferns in the understory and less moss coating tree trunks. Look for the tiny pink blossoms of star flower (*Trientalis latifolia*) along the trail.

As you near the valley floor, you reach the Olema Valley Trail and turn left. The trail descends steeply for nearly half a mile and soon crosses a tributary of Olema Creek. You return to Five Brooks along this fault-line route, the stream meandering on a gentle course to your right. At the Five Brooks mill pond, turn right and circle the south side of the pond, looking for birds in the willows and alders that edge the water.

The San Andreas fault cuts directly through the shallow trough of Olema Valley. Movement along the fault formed the waterways that lie at both ends of the valley—Tomales Bay and Bolinas Lagoon. Fault zones often create jumbled topography, and Olema Valley's uplifted and folded hills and ridges are no exception. The small lakes, or "sag ponds," that spring up along the valley's floor are also typical of fault zones.

Stewart Trail to Wildcat Camp

Trip 27

The Stewart Trail is the only trail in the vicinity open to bikes, and is cyclists' only option to reach Wildcat Camp. A wide, well-graded route in a shady forest, the trail offers great views on both the west and east sides of Inverness Ridge—of Olema Valley and of the coast. Hikers and equestrians might find that combining the Stewart Trail with some of the numerous other trails that lead to the coast makes for a more interesting route.

Distance: 12.8 miles
Type: Out-and-back
Difficulty: Strenuous
Facilities: Toilets, water at Five Brooks Trailhead; toilet at Wildcat Camp, no potable water
Regulations: Horses and bikes allowed on Stewart Trail; permit required for overnight camping at Wildcat Camp.

Begin on the wide trail that skirts the mill pond, passing the Rift Zone Trail and arriving at a junction with the Stewart and Olema Valley trails 0.1 mile from your car. Turn right on the Stewart Trail. After an immediate and brief descent, you climb gently through a lush forest of Douglas-fir, bay laurel, big-leaf maple, hazelnut, and alder, with ferns and poison oak in the understory.

You pass the Greenpicker Trail after 0.9 mile and follow the Stewart Trail as it swings sharply to the left and continues on a gradual climb up Inverness Ridge. The wide trail—an old ranch road that the Army improved during World

War II—is broad enough to accommodate the horses, bicyclists, and hikers that you are likely to encounter on pleasant weekends.

A steep and wooded ravine drops below the trail, where a small waterway descends to Olema Creek; look out across Olema Valley to the rounded swells of Bolinas Ridge. A light canopy of trees extends over the trail, sprinkling it with shadows and keeping you cool.

Pass the Ridge Trail on the left as it begins its way south along the crest of Inverness Ridge, and stay on the Stewart Trail, reaching the level, open meadow at Firtop less than a mile later (3.6 miles from the trailhead). The trail continues across Firtop and leaves the meadow on a steep descent, back in the forest. After less than half a mile, you meet the Ridge Trail again on the left, and a short spur trail on your right leads to the Greenpicker Trail.

The Stewart Trail continues its westward course to the coast. Beneath the dirt track, the remnants of pavement appear, reminding you of the history of this land. At the top of a slight rise, you have your first views of the coast. The rest of the route to Wildcat Camp winds down the western slope of Inverness Ridge on a gentle-to-moderate descent, passing Old Out Road and the Glen and Coast trails before reaching the camp.

Bikes must return on the Stewart Trail, but hikers and equestrians can explore other routes back to the trailhead.

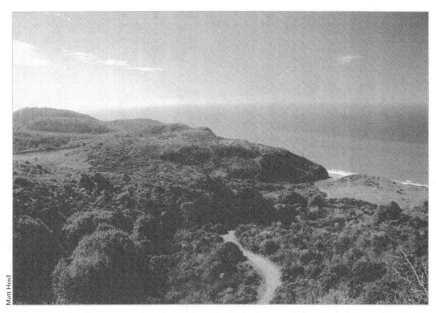

Matt Heid

The Stewart Trail with Wildcat Camp below and the coast beyond

Wildcat Camp and Beach via the Greenpicker Trail

The transition from forested ridge to open coast is the highlight of this trip. You follow the narrow Greenpicker Trail up the ridge to reach high littoral bluffs. Exhilarating views accompany your descent to the coast through fragrant coastal scrub and spring-blooming ceanothus and iris. You can chose between two return routes.

Distance: 11.6 miles returning on the Stewart Trail; 13.1 miles returning on Old Out Road and Alamea Trail
Difficulty: Strenuous
Type: Loop
Facilities: Toilets, water at Five Brooks Trailhead
Regulations: Horses allowed; bikes allowed on Stewart Trail; no dogs

The wide trail from the parking area skirts the mill pond and passes the Rift Zone Trail to arrive at a junction with the Stewart and Olema Valley trails, 0.1 mile from the trailhead. Turn right on the Stewart Trail, an old ranch road, and make an immediate and brief descent. You then climb gently through a lush forest of Douglas-fir, bay laurel, big-leaf maple, hazelnut, and alder, above a deep creek ravine.

After 0.9 mile from the trailhead, you leave the Stewart Trail and pick up the narrow Greenpicker Trail. Lined with lush vegetation, Greenpicker is slightly shorter than the Stewart Trail, although a bit steeper. Tanbark oak, bay laurel, and Douglas-fir trees overshadow masses of huckleberry bushes, and cow parsnip, blackberry, and sword ferns crowd the edges of the path.

You enter a dense corridor of Douglas-firs as you near Firtop, and the trail widens and levels. The lush understory disappears, brown trunks stretch to towering heights, and dry needles cushion the trail. At the first junction, go straight to make a 0.1-mile detour to Firtop. Otherwise, veer right to continue on the Greenpicker Trail, which wraps around the high knoll of Firtop. Just 0.7 mile farther, you reach a junction with a spur trail, which offers the option of connecting to the Stewart or Ridge trails. Stay right on Greenpicker, and descend gradually through subtly changing vegetation—coyote bush becomes more frequent, often joined by wild cucumber—indicating the increasing proximity of the coast.

One mile beyond the last junction (4.4 miles from the trailhead), you turn left on the wide Glen Camp Loop Trail, and follow its level course for a short 0.2 mile. Pass the Glen Trail and veer right on the Coast/Glen Spur South. The path borders a marshy swale, filled with rushes and horsetails, and reaches the Coast Trail in 0.4 mile, where you veer left. Bordered by young Douglas-fir, coyote bush, blackberry, and coffeeberry, this narrow trail quickly emerges on the bluff overlooking the blue-green ocean, glistening in the sun or fading into fog. Smells of the ocean and coastal scrub are pungent, and springtime blossoms of morning glory and lupine grace the bluffs. You have views south of Wildcat Lake and of Double Point.

At the junction with the Stewart Trail (5.9 miles from the trailhead), you can turn left and head back up the ridge on the wide, smooth trail. Or turn right to reach Wildcat Camp and other return options.

To return via the Stewart Trail:
The exposed Stewart Trail climbs up the ridge, bordered by bay laurel, young Douglas-fir, coyote bush, chamise, wild cucumber, sticky monkeyflower, and cow parsnip. If you've had enough climbing once you've reached the crest, turn right on the Ridge Trail to avoid a steep climb to Firtop on the Stewart Trail and to shorten your route slightly. A delightful narrow path, rangy elderberry and huckleberry bushes often spill onto the Ridge Trail, and sunlight wafts through tall Douglas-firs. The trail may be muddy in spring. After half a mile, you veer left and soon rejoin the Stewart Trail, which descends gradually to return to the trailhead in 2.7 miles.

To return via Old Out Road and the Alamea Trail:
If you turn right at the junction with the Stewart and Coast trails (5.9 miles from the trailhead), you head downhill for 0.7 mile to Wildcat Camp, situated on a low bluff behind the beach. The camp is a good spot for a picnic, and a small path at the southern end of the camp, near a small willow-lined stream, leads to the beach. Wildcat Beach stretches for 2 miles, limited on the south by Alamere Falls and on the north by steep cliffs that drop to the water.

Follow the Coast Trail as it passes through Wildcat Camp and continues south, inland from the immediate bluffs. After just 0.2 mile from the camp, you pass the Ocean Lake Loop Trail and climb gently on the Coast Trail through tall cow parsnip and ceanothus. Shortly beyond the shores of reed-lined Wildcat Lake, turn left on Old Out Road. The old ranch road (bits and pieces of asphalt break through the dirt in places) heads up Inverness Ridge, mostly shaded by Douglas-fir. After 1.1 miles, you veer left on the Alamea Trail and continue climbing for a short while until the trail levels and then meets the Ridge Trail, 1.5 miles from Old Out Road.

Either way you turn on the Ridge Trail, you soon will join the Stewart Trail. The shorter route back to the trailhead is to the right: follow the singletrack Ridge Trail for about 0.4 mile, carefully avoiding the stinging nettle and the muddy patches that plague the trail in spring. Turn left at the first junction to meet the Stewart Trail very shortly, where you turn right and follow the wide dirt road 2.8 miles back to Five Brooks.

Shuttle Trip to Palomarin

This hike is worth the extra effort it takes to arrange a shuttle trip. Begin along the San Andreas fault in Olema Valley, climb through dense forest to exquisite views of the coast, and complete the trip on open bluffs. Bass Lake, the best swimming spot around, is just a short detour off the main route.

Distance: 7.7 miles one-way; 8.7 with side trip to Bass Lake
Type: Shuttle
Difficulty: Moderate to strenuous
Facilities: Toilets, water at Five Brooks Trailhead; toilets at Palomarin Trailhead
Regulations: Horses allowed; no bikes; no dogs

Begin on the wide trail from the parking area and shortly veer left at the circular cement horse fountain in the grassy field. Pick up a small trail around the mill pond. Turn left at the tip of the pond on the wide Olema Valley Trail, beneath a thick, leafy cover of alder, bay laurel, and hazelnut. This trail is often muddy in wet weather. After crossing a creek, you begin a fairly steep half-mile climb. At 1.4 miles from the trailhead, turn right on the Bolema Trail, which heads up the western slope of Inverness Ridge. Douglas-fir and tanbark oak shade the steady mile-long climb to the junction with the Ridge and Lake Ranch trails.

Cross the Ridge Trail and head southwest on the wide Lake Ranch Trail, an old road that led to the ranch of the same name. Summertime fog drip from the towering Douglas-firs and winter rain often create muddy patches, and branches and needles felled in storms litter the trail in winter. You soon reach Mud Lake, ringed by oak and Douglas-fir trees; a grassy, poppy-covered hillside rises from one shore. The trail climbs gently out of the small basin.

A rich, evergreen fragrance drifts through the air, and the moist forest supports an understory of coffeeberry, huckleberry, elderberry, and ferns. You begin to descend the eastern slope of Inverness Ridge, the grade tempered by wide switchbacks. The soft dirt trail is alternately exposed and shaded, and you can catch great views of the Pacific through mossy branches. As you near the Coast Trail, firs cast shade over the large stands of coffeeberry, thimbleberry, and blackberry; leaves hang delicately from abundant hazelnut bushes, wild cucumber

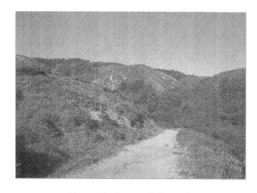

Coast Trail near Palomarin

sprawls over the scrub thickets, and cow parsnip grows profusely. Poison oak is abundant, although the trail is wide enough that you can avoid it.

You reach the junction with the Coast Trail, 5.5 miles from the trailhead. To detour to Bass Lake (a 1-mile round trip), turn right and descend gradually beneath a shady canopy of alders and willows. Emerging once again into the open, you see the tranquil lake on the left beyond a coastal-scrub–covered slope. At the far end of the lake, a short trail leads to a grassy gathering spot for pic-nickers and swimmers. A dip in the lake on warm days is an exquisite pleasure.

To continue directly to the Palomarin Trailhead from the Lake Ranch/Coast trails junction, turn left and ascend slightly past two small lily-pad–decorated ponds to the right of the trail. Look for killdeer, swallows, and red winged black-birds. The trail becomes rocky and narrower and, after passing between high rock walls, emerges to ocean views and descends a dry coastal slope, lined by young Douglas-firs.

The remainder of the hike follows the exposed bluff, traversing wide gullies cut by streams, with excellent views of Bolinas Point to the south and Abalone Point to the north. Seep monkeyflower blooms in spring among watercress and horsetail in moist ravines. Fragrant coastal scrub covers the hillsides, interspersed with brilliant spring and summer wildflowers—orange sticky monkeyflower, red and yellow Indian paintbrush, blue lupine, yellow buttercups, and iris. Just before the Palomarin Trailhead, you enter a eucalyptus grove, where South End Ranch used to stand.

Shuttle Trip to Arch Rock via the Greenpicker and Coast trails; return through Bear Valley

A great all-day hike, these trails take you from dense forest to open coast to lush creekside. You'll see spring wildflowers and exceptional coastal views. Arch Rock and Millers Point on the coast are great pic-nic and whale-watching spots.

Distance: 11 miles one-way
Type: Shuttle
Difficulty: Strenuous
Facilities: Toilets, water at Five Brooks and Bear Valley trailheads; toilets at Divide Meadow (9.1 miles)
Regulations: No dogs; bikes allowed on Bear Valley Trail from Glen Trail to trailhead

A wide trail rings the mill pond at the trailhead. Circle the pond on the right, passing the Rift Zone Trail, and at the far end of the pond, 0.1 mile from your car, you turn right on the Stewart Trail. (The Olema Valley Trail goes left, heading south through the valley.) After an immediate and brief descent on the Stewart Trail, an old ranch road, you climb gently through a lush forest of Douglas-fir, bay laurel, big-leaf maple, hazelnut, and alder, with ferns and poison oak as vibrant undergrowth. The trail rings the deep ravine of a creek that descends the ridge to Olema Creek.

After 0.9 mile from the trailhead, you leave the old ranch road for the narrow Greenpicker Trail, closed to bikes. Although steeper than the Stewart Trail, Greenpicker is slightly shorter and provides a more varied route, densely lined with lush vegetation. Tanbark oaks, bay laurels, and Douglas-firs overshadow masses of huckleberry bushes, and cow parsnip, blackberry, and sword ferns crowd the edges of the path.

You enter a dense corridor of Douglas-fir as you near Firtop, and the trail widens and levels. The lush understory disappears, brown trunks stretch to towering heights, and dry needles cushion the trail. At the first junction, veer right to continue on the Greenpicker Trail, which wraps around the high knoll of Firtop. Now beyond the dry corridor of Douglas-fir, the vegetation returns, and you descend through a quiet forest that is a vivid collage of green in spring. Just 0.7 mile beyond the last junction, you reach an intersection with a spur trail, which offers the option of connecting to the Stewart or Ridge trails. Stay right on Greenpicker, and descend gradually through subtly changing vegetation—coyote bush becomes more frequent, often joined by wild cucumber—indicating the increasing proximity of the coast.

A mile farther (4.4 miles from the trailhead), you turn left on the wide Glen Camp Loop Trail, and follow its level course for a short 0.2 mile. Pass the right-branching Glen Trail and veer right on the Coast/Glen Spur South. The path borders a marshy swale, filled with rushes and horsetails, and takes you, in less than half a mile, to the Coast Trail. Turn right and head west on a narrow path bordered by a thicket of blackberry, poison oak, and coyote bush. After 0.6 mile from the junction, you meet the spur trail from the Glen Trail in a grassy expanse dotted with coyote bush.

Continue west on the Coast Trail, which soon begins to descend gradually. You emerge from high shrubs to fabulous ocean views, on a coastal hillside swathed with spring wildflowers in bright yellows, blues, and oranges. You soon reach a small knoll just to the left of the trail, a good rest and view spot. The trail then descends more steeply, eroded in patches, and reaches Millers Point and the coast. It curves to the right and heads north to the bluff across from Arch Rock.

You pass through lush vegetation, sprinkled with the rounded white umbels of cow parsnip, and the white flowers or red fruits of elderberry. A wooden bridge, flanked by alders, crosses the mouth of Coast Creek. The trail rises to a junction with a path that leads 0.1 mile to Arch Rock. Turn left for a worthwhile 0.1-mile side trip to the dramatic promontory above the sea, where you can look down on the rocky beach below. You'll have clear-day views from Chimney Rock to Double Point and out to the Farallon Islands.

Return to the junction and veer right for 0.1 mile to reach the Bear Valley Trail. You will have come 7 miles from the trailhead at this point and can make an easy return along this wide, multi-use trail.

The trail soon enters the shade of alders and follows the lush bed of Coast Creek. You pass the Glen Trail 0.9 mile from the coast, a possible route back to Five Brooks. You soon ascend the gentle slope of Divide Meadow, where oaks provide a bit of shade on the broad expanse, a perfect spot for a rest. But you are only 1.6 miles from the Bear Valley Trailhead, your final destination, which you will reach after a brief descent and a level, shaded course along Bear Valley Creek.

PALOMARIN TRAILS AND BEACHES

A dirt road crosses the southern tip of the Point Reyes peninsula, heading west over the coastal mesa, past a Coast Guard radio facility, a beef cattle ranch, and the Point Reyes Bird Observatory to reach the Palomarin Trailhead. The southernmost trailhead in the park, Palomarin is an entry point for unbeatable hikes along the coastal bluff all the way to Wildcat Camp and Beach, past the only freshwater lakes in the park (great swimming!). A mile-long trail to Palomarin Beach begins about a mile before the trailhead.

Driving Directions: From Hwy. 1 at 4.5 miles north of Stinson Beach and 9 miles south of Olema, turn west at the often unsigned Bolinas turnoff. Continue 1.7 miles to Mesa Rd. and turn right. Mesa Rd. ends at the Palomarin Trailhead, 1.8 miles beyond the Point Reyes Bird Observatory.
Facilities: Toilet at trailhead.

South End Ranch

South End Ranch once lay among the eucalyptus trees at the Palomarin trailhead. A functioning dairy ranch for several decades, the brushy landscape eventually proved too difficult to continue grazing. The Christ Church of the Golden Rule bought it in 1950 and created a self-contained community with homes, barns, schools, and a nursery business. In 1963, the church sold the land to the National Park Service, and only a former school building remains today as the Point Reyes Bird Observatory.

Note: The Crystal Lake Trail is no longer maintained by the National Park Service and is overgrown with poison oak and stinging nettle. The spur trails to Double Point and Alamere Falls, although mentioned in this guidebook, are also unmaintained and overgrown.

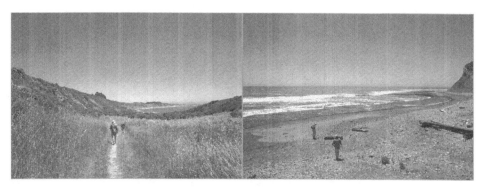

Trail to Palomarin Beach   Palomarin Beach

This rocky beach between Double and Duxberry points offers great tidepooling.

Driving Directions: From Hwy. 1 at 4.5 miles north of Stinson Beach and 9 miles south of Olema, turn west at the often unsigned Bolinas turnoff. Continue 1.7 miles to Mesa Rd. and turn right. Palomarin Beach parking is about a half mile beyond the Point Reyes Bird Observatory.

Facilities: None

Regulations: No camping, no overnight parking, no dogs

The Beach: The southernmost beach in Point Reyes National Seashore, Palomarin is accessed on a wide, 1-mile trail down a hillside overtaken by eucalyptus and scotch broom. High, eroding cliffs rise behind a narrow strip of sand, and the rocky beach provides good habitat for tidepools.

Coast Trail to Bass Lake, Alamere Falls, Wildcat Camp

Trip 31

Seals, swimming, whales, wildflowers, and a waterfall! This trip along the Coast Trail offers numerous activities and destinations, depending on your stamina. Picnic and swim at freshwater Bass Lake, look for wildlife from coastal promontories, and visit dramatic Alamere Falls and the ocean. With a camping permit, you can spend a night at Wildcat Camp.

Distance: 2.7 miles one-way to Bass Lake; 4 miles one-way to Double Point; 4 miles one-way to Alamere Falls; 5.7 miles one-way to Wildcat Camp

Type: Out-and-back

Facilities: Toilets at Palomarin trailhead and Wildcat Camp; no potable water at Wildcat Camp

Regulations: No dogs; no bikes

The Coast Trail begins from the dirt parking lot on a short wooden staircase. The old ranch road, lined with sprawling blackberry and wild cucumber vines, quickly enters a eucalyptus grove and then emerges onto open coastal bluffs. Coyote bush releases its distinct spicy fragrance, and orange sticky monkeyflower, red and yellow Indian paintbrush, blue lupine, and yellow bush lupine add bright spots of color when in bloom.

Following the coastline, the trail wanders in and out of wide gullies cut by small streams, where seep monkeyflower blooms in spring among watercress and horsetail. Cow parsnip, iris, buttercups, blackberry, and ferns enliven the moist hillside ravines. Excellent views accompany you on these exposed coastal bluffs:

Bolinas Point lies to the south, and to the north the coastline stretches to Abalone and Double points. Far below, waves crash onto the narrow, pebbly beach at the foot of steep cliffs.

The trail soon begins a brief switchback up a dry slope, leaving the coast behind. Young Douglas-firs encroach on both sides and will soon turn this open stretch into a shaded one. In spring, bright-green new growth extends from the branch tips. As you near the crest, high walls enclose the rocky trail.

On a gentle descent, you pass two small lily-pad-decorated ponds to the left of the trail—look for killdeer, swallows, and red-winged blackbirds—and a junction with the Lake Ranch Trail, 2.2 miles from the trailhead. Beyond, the trail levels and then descends gradually beneath a shady canopy of alders and willows. Emerging from the trees, you see tranquil Bass Lake on the left of the trail. At the far end of the lake, 2.7 miles from the trailhead, a short trail leads to a grassy spot where picnickers and swimmers gather on warm days.

The freshwater coastal lakes in this region are the result of a nearly 5-mile-long landslide, extending from Double Point to Bear Valley. Large chunks of flinty Monterey shale, the rock that overlays the peninsula's granite bedrock here, have broken off. Tilting and contorting as they slid into the ocean, the rocks created these small lakes.

Now under the cover of Douglas-fir and lined by coffeeberry and ceanothus bushes, the trail climbs a moderate incline and passes the unmaintained Crystal Lake Trail, overgrown with poison oak and stinging nettle. You soon emerge from the trees and look down upon Pelican Lake, with the open coast beyond. Double Point, a large shale promontory jutting into the Pacific, rises ahead of you. Follow the trail as it descends gently around the lake, following signs with the symbol of a hiker, to a pair of small paths (3.7 miles from the trailhead). The

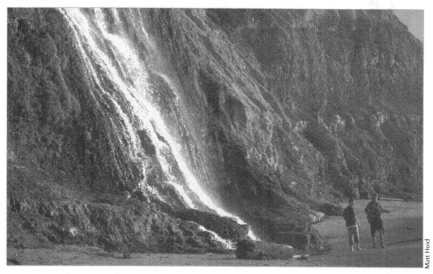

Alamere Falls

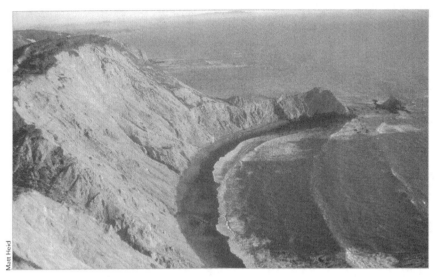

Double Point

first one leads to Double Point in about a half mile. The park does not maintain the path and discourages visitors from using it. If you do, stay back from the cliff edges, which are unstable and dangerous, and respect the animals that reside on the beach and rocks below. Double Point is a sensitive wildlife habitat for harbor seals, sea otters, and murres.

Just beyond the turnoff to Double Point, a small path heads to the coast at Alamere Falls, The narrow, overgrown path is also unmaintained by the park, and reaches the beach by way of a rocky scramble down a steep and eroding cliff-side. The park advises hikers who want to visit the falls to continue on the Coast Trail to Wildcat Beach and backtrack for about a mile on the sand.

Past the spur to Alamere Falls, the Coast Trail continues north and descends to the lush bed of Alamere Creek, where you cross a wooden bridge shaded by alders and willows. At 4.3 miles from the trailhead, you reach a junction where the Ocean Lake Loop Trail veers left. This exceptionally scenic trail traces the coastline west of Ocean Lake, providing views of it and Wildcat Lake, and the sweep of coast north all the way to Chimney Rock. Although just about the same length as the Coast Trail, the Ocean Lake Trail has a few more ups and downs. The Coast Trail stays inland, lined by fragrant ceanothus, and soon passes Old Out Road, a possible route to the ridgetop and the Five Brooks Trailhead. After 1.1 miles, the Coast and Ocean Lake Loop trails converge, and descend briefly to Wildcat Camp.

After exploring Wildcat Beach, you can take the Stewart or Old Out trails to the Five Brooks Trailhead, or retrace your steps to the Palomarin Trailhead, unless you have a camping permit for Wildcat, the best option of all! (See Backpack Trips 4 and 7, pages 203, 205–206.)

Coast and Ridge Loop

This diverse loop travels exposed coastal bluffs, shaded Douglas-fir forests, and peaceful ridgetop meadows. You'll have exhilarating views along the coast, climb to the top of Inverness Ridge, and then head south along its crest to return. The loop finishes with a short stint on Mesa Road, the dirt road you drove on to reach the trailhead. The open bluffs offer no protection from the elements—dress accordingly to insulate yourself from sun, wind, or fog.

Distance: 11.2 miles
Type: Loop
Facilities: Toilets at trailhead; no water
Regulations: Horses allowed; no bikes or dogs

The Coast Trail begins from the dirt parking lot on a short wooden staircase. Sprawling blackberry and wild cucumber vines line the old ranch road as it passes through a eucalyptus grove and then emerges onto open coastal bluffs. The smell of the sea mixes with the spicy fragrance of coyote bush, and orange sticky monkeyflower, red and yellow Indian paintbrush, blue lupine, and yellow bush lupine bloom on the hillside in season. The trail follows the coastline, in and out of wide stream gullies where seep monkeyflower blooms in spring among watercress and horsetail. In the moist hillside ravines, cow parsnip, iris, buttercups, and blackberry thrive. You'll have excellent views from the exposed coastal bluffs: Bolinas Point lies to the south and Abalone Point to the north. Far below, waves crash onto the narrow, pebbly beach at the foot of steep cliffs.

Among young Douglas-firs, the trail begins a brief switchback up a dry slope to leave the coast behind. As you near the crest, high walls enclose the rocky trail. At the first junction (2.2 miles from the trailhead) you turn right and follow the wide, grassy Lake Ranch Trail, once a farm road. Cow parsnip intersperses large stands of coffeeberry, leaves hang delicately from abundant hazelnut bushes, and thimbleberry, blackberry, and wild cucumber grow along the trail. Poison oak is abundant, but doesn't encroach on the wide trail.

The soft dirt trail climbs gentle switchbacks to the ridge, alternately exposed and shaded, allowing great views of the Pacific between mossy Douglas-fir branches. Fog frequently visits these coastal hillsides, keeping the forest moist. Seasonal storms bring high winds that litter the trail with small branches and needles. Coffeeberry, huckleberry, elderberry, and ferns create a rich understory, and a strong evergreen fragrance fills the air. At Mud Lake, the trail descends and wraps around the marshy pond's northwest shore, where a grassy, poppy-covered hillside meets the lake.

Turn right on the Ridge Trail and head southeast along the crest of forested Inverness Ridge for about 4 miles. Sunlight spills through Douglas-firs in patches, and ferns carpet the ground. Vibrant green moss lines the soft trail, cluttered with small branches. Mud sometimes oozes across the trail, but you can avoid the worst of it.

Lake Ranch

The Coast Trail route once led to Lake Ranch, where a ranch house stood near these two small ponds along the trail. In the 1940s, following rumors of oil, the ranch owner granted an oil lease to the National Exploration Company to drill on his land, but the venture met with little success. In another attempt at financial gain, he sold his timber rights on Inverness Ridge to the Sweet Lumber Company, which logged the Douglas-firs until 1963. The Sweet family bought the ranch and began work on a housing development at Lake Ranch in the 1960s. The Park Service terminated the development when it finally purchased the land in 1971.

Once you pass the Teixeira Trail, the ocean's presence becomes tangible in the subtly changing vegetation and salty breeze: the wind picks up, poison oak reappears, cow parsnip and wild cucumber reclaim prominence, and sticky monkeyflower mingles with elderberry and huckleberry. You pass small, bushy Douglas-fir, open swards of grasses, and bright-orange springtime poppies along the trail. As you descend gently, views of the coast periodically peek through trees, tall bush lupine, and coyote bush. To the east, densely forested Olema Ridge slopes toward the town of Bolinas, with Bolinas Lagoon and Bolinas Ridge in the distance.

As the descent steepens, you can see waves crashing against the coastline. Watch out for abundant poison oak. After a brief but steep downhill, from which you see Mesa Road winding toward Palomarin, you arrive at the open dirt road. Surprisingly rich vegetation lines the road—iris, ceanothus, and thimbleberry—and buckeye and bay laurel grow in the riparian ravine. As you return to the trailhead, enjoy great coastal views beyond the dense coastal scrub on the bluffs.

BACKPACKING

Nothing compares to spending a night under the stars (even if they're obscured by fog). With four campgrounds and 32,000 acres of wilderness, and only 30 miles from the urban San Francisco Bay Area, Point Reyes National Seashore offers numerous possibilities for overnight escapes.

You must plan ahead for a camping trip at Point Reyes. All campsites require an advance reservation, which you can make up to three months in advance (to the day). Campers quickly snatch up reservations for weekends and holidays throughout the year, and summer weekdays also fill up early. To reserve, call (415) 663-8054 between 9 A.M. and 2 P.M., Monday through Friday; come to Bear Valley Visitor Center in person, seven days a week; or fax your reservation to (415) 464-5149 using the park fax form.

Phone reservations require payment by credit card, due at the time you make the reservation. Permits cost $12 per night per site for sites that accommodate up to six people, $25 for seven to 14 people, and $35 for 15 to 25 people. On January 1, 2005, fees will be $15 (up to six people), $30 (seven to 14 people), and $40 (15 to 25 people). No refunds are given for any reason, including weather and illness.

Pick up your permit at the visitor center before beginning your trip. If you arrive after the visitor center has closed, you will find your permit in the after-hours box on the information board in front of the building.

Campsites have a picnic table, food locker, and charcoal grill. (No wood fires are allowed in the park; you must use the charcoal grill or bring a gas stove.) Every campground has a pit toilet and a water faucet; water from the faucet is potable except at Wildcat Camp, where you must treat it with chlorine, iodine tablets, a filter, or by boiling for one minute. Do not drink untreated water from streams or lakes.

All camps are all close enough to trailheads to make one a dayhike destination.

BACKPACKING CAMP REGULATIONS
- Store food in storage lockers to protect it from animals
- Wash dishes away from water spigots
- Do not feed wildlife
- Pack out all trash
- No wood fires; use charcoal in the grill or a gas stove; no collection of downed wood; driftwood fires allowed on sandy beaches with a permit
- Respect your camp neighbors: observe quiet hours, from sunset to sunrise
- Camping outside designated campsites or without a permit is illegal
- No dogs or other pets allowed on any trails or in any of the campgrounds
- Four-night per visit limit; maximum of 30 nights per year

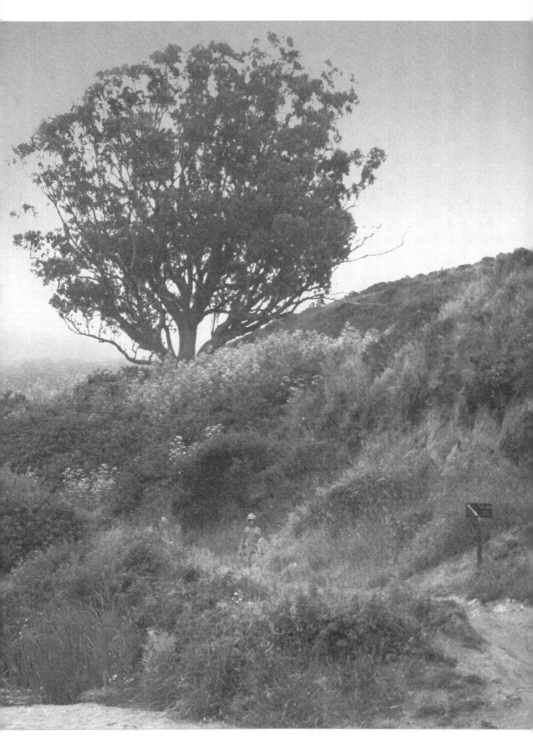

Trail from Santa Maria Beach to Coast Camp

- Maximum number of stock or horses is eight per campground; animals must be tied to hitch rails
- No firearms or fireworks

BACKPACKING CAMPS

Sky Camp

Perched on the coastal slopes of Mt. Wittenberg, Sky Camp looks out on a spectacular view of Drakes Bay, the coast, Chimney Rock, and the lighthouse point. A view, that is, when the coast and peninsula below aren't obscured by fog; but when they are, another bonus of Sky Camp's location reveals itself—at 1025 feet, the camp often escapes the thick white tide that rolls over the coast.

Sky Camp is on the site of the former Z Ranch, first run by the Wittenbergs, for whom Mt. Wittenberg is named. Grazing kept the shrubs and young Douglas-firs on the hillsides at bay, and open pastureland surrounded the ranch. The only reminder of the ranch today is the spring that provides water for the camp.

Most campsites are off the main trail, tucked among shrubs of coyote bush and small stands of Douglas-firs. They have excellent views and a secluded feeling. The shortest route to Sky Camp is from the Sky Trailhead on Limantour Road (see Limantour Road, pages 120–144).

Details:
- 12 sites, including one group site
- Hitch rail and horse water trough
- Bicycle access via Sky Trail only
- 1.3 miles from the nearest trailhead (Sky Trailhead)
- 3 miles from Bear Valley via the Mt. Wittenberg and Sky trails

Coast Camp

Just a few steps from Santa Maria Beach and a short walk from Sculptured, Secret, and Limantour beaches, Coast Camp is a great place to spend a night or two and explore these magical beaches by day. A low, sandy ridge protects the camp from ocean breezes, and the view from the camp stretches up the slopes of Inverness Ridge.

Coast Camp is on the site of long-abandoned U Ranch, the only remnant of which is a large eucalyptus tree that stands above the small path to the beach, marking the location of the camp from miles away. North of the camp, ranchers grew hay on the flat marine terrace.

Several campsites border the Coast Trail, which passes through the camp; more secluded sites are dispersed on the small knoll above the trail. You can reach Coast Camp directly from the Point Reyes hostel trailhead, from Limantour Beach, or from the Sky Trailhead. Routes vary in difficulty and distance (see Limantour Road, pages 120–144).

Details:
- 14 sites, including 2 group sites
- Hitch rail
- Bicycle access via Coast Trail only
- 1.5 miles by walking on the beach from the southern Limantour parking lot
- 1.8 miles (slight uphill, then descent) via the Laguna and Fire Lane trails from the Point Reyes hostel trailhead
- 2.8 miles (level) on Coast Trail from the Point Reyes hostel trailhead (bike route)
- 7.9 miles on Coast Trail from Wildcat Camp

Glen Camp

Surrounded by towering Douglas-firs and tucked in a protected valley, Glen Camp is one of the seashore's most peaceful and out-of-the-way overnight retreats. Until the 1920s, Glen Ranch operated in this open meadow, although no ranch buildings remain.

Campsites are widely dispersed, some in the meadow and others sheltered by trees. An overnight at Glen Camp offers possibilities of numerous dayhikes—to Wildcat Beach, Arch Rock, and Firtop.

The shortest route to the camp (4.6 miles) is from Bear Valley; bicyclists must approach from the Five Brooks Trailhead, which is also a nice route for hikers, although slightly longer. (See Bear Valley and Five Brooks trailheads sections for detailed descriptions of the hikes to the camp.)

Details:
- 12 sites
- Bicycle access from Five Brooks only
- No groups, horses, or pack animals
- 2.7 miles to Wildcat Beach and Camp
- 4.6 miles from Bear Valley on Bear Valley, Glen, and Glen Camp Loop trails
- 6.4 miles from Five Brooks on Stewart and Glen trails (bike route)
- 4.9 miles from Five Brooks on Greenpicker and Glen Camp Loop trails

Wildcat Camp

Falling asleep to the sound of the waves on Wildcat Beach, awakening to a landscape ensconced in fog, and walking the beach as the low mist peels back to reveal a sparkling day are some of the great treasures of camping at Point Reyes. The most remote camp in the park, Wildcat Camp sits on an open coastal bluff, 5.7 miles from the nearest trailhead. A short trail from the camp leads to Wildcat Beach, which stretches for about 2 miles, with Alamere Falls at its southern end.

In the 19th century, Wildcat Ranch was known for the butter it produced as well as its picturesque location. During World War II, the U.S. Army built a military reservation on a cliff above the ranch site. A stand of eucalyptus trees at

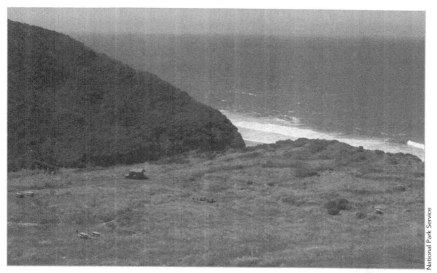

Wildcat Camp

the campground is a reminder of this history, and the Stewart Trail, a former ranch road improved by the military, remains as one of the routes to the camp.

Wildcat is the smallest of the four camps in the park and is the only one that does not provide potable water.

Details:
- Seven sites, including three group sites; three of the individual sites accommodate only up to four people
- Bicycle access from Five Brooks only
- 5.7 miles from Palomarin Trailhead on Coast Trail
- 6.6 miles from Bear Valley Trailhead on Bear Valley, Glen, and Coast trails
- 6.4 miles from Five Brooks Trailhead on Stewart Trail (bike route)

Closest Entry Points

For a campers getting a late start, families with kids, or anyone looking for the least taxing trip possible, Sky and Coast camps offer the shortest access hikes. The Sky Trailhead is as close as you can get to any of the camps—1.3 miles up an initially steep incline, and then a fairly level trail. Coast Camp is 1.4 miles if you begin at the Limantour parking lot and take the level beach route to the camp. From the Laguna Trailhead, the route is a hillier 1.8 miles, and from the Point Reyes hostel, a level 2.8-mile trail leads to Coast Camp.

Bike Trips

Bikes have 2 options: the Coast Trail from the Point Reyes hostel trailhead to Coast Camp (2.8 miles) or the Stewart Trail from Five Brooks Trailhead to Wildcat Camp (6.5 miles).

The following represent a few possible routes for a backpack trip in Point Reyes. Most of these routes are described in detail in other sections of this book, so you'll just find a brief overview here; routes between camps, not described in other sections, are given in more detail here.

One-night Weekend at the Beach

Wildcat Camp via the Coast Trail from Palomarin

5.7 MILES

This is a fairly level route along the Coast Trail from the Palomarin Trailhead. A few ups and downs will make you feel like you've earned a swim in Bass Lake, about half way to Wildcat Camp. You'll have great views along these coastal bluffs.

Coast Camp via the beach from Limantour Trailhead

1.4 MILES

From the southernmost parking area at Limantour Beach, take the narrow trail to the beach and follow the sand for 1.4 miles to the landmark eucalyptus tree on the bluff. A short path leads from the beach to Coast Camp.

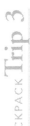

Coast Camp via the Coast Trail from Laguna Trailhead near Point Reyes hostel

1.8 MILES

From the Laguna Trailhead along the Point Reyes hostel road, the Laguna Trail makes a gradual climb to the Fire Lane Trail, which you then follow on a moderate descent to Coast Camp, taking in views of Drakes Bay and the Pacific.

Wildcat and Coast camps

First day: Palomarin to Wildcat Camp, 5.7 miles
Second day: Wildcat Camp to Coast Camp on the Coast Trail, 7.9 miles
Third day: Coast Camp to Limantour or Point Reyes hostel, 1.4 or 2.8 miles

This trip requires a car shuttle since you begin at the Palomarin Trailhead and end at Limantour Beach or the Point Reyes hostel.

Follow trip number 1 above, Palomarin to Wildcat Camp. The next day, head north from Wildcat Camp and turn left in 0.7 mile on the Coast Trail. Climb the coastal bluff and turn left at the next junction to continue on the Coast Trail. Pass a spur trail and descend gradually and then more steeply to the coast, where the trail heads north (right). Just before a junction with the Bear Valley Trail, veer left on a 0.1-mile path to Arch Rock for dramatic views.

Return to the Coast Trail and continue north along the coastal bluff for 4.2 miles to Coast Camp. Listen for sea lions off of Point Resistance, look for pelagic birds, take in impressive views of Drakes Bay and Chimney Rock, and enjoy the sweet fragrance of ceanothus in springtime.

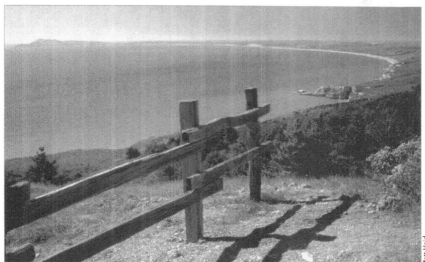

Matt Heid

Coast Trail south of Arch Rock

From Coast Camp, if your shuttle car is at the Limantour Trailhead, reach it via a 1.4-mile walk along the beach; if your car is at the Point Reyes hostel trailhead, continue on the Coast Trail for 2.8 miles.

If you want a shorter hike on your first day, you can do the above trip in reverse, beginning at Coast Camp. Then continue down the coast to Wildcat Camp and at end Palomarin.

First day: Limantour or Point Reyes hostel to Coast Camp, 1.4 or 2.8 miles
Second day: Coast Camp to Wildcat Camp on the Coast Trail, 7.9 miles
Third day: Wildcat Camp to Palomarin, 5.7 miles

Two-night Weekend Ridge to Coast, Shuttle or Loop

BACKPACK Trip 5 | Sky and Coast camps

SHUTTLE OR LOOP

First day: Sky Trailhead to Sky Camp, 1.3 miles
Second day: Sky Camp to Coast Camp, 4.2 miles
Third day: Coast Camp to Limantour Trailhead, 1.4 miles, or Point Reyes hostel trailhead, 2.8 miles (shuttle); to Sky Trailhead, 4.1 miles

Sky Camp is a short walk on the Sky Trail (with a steep but brief climb). The second day your trail is level and descending, along the crest of Inverness Ridge and then down the coastal slope to Coast Camp.

After a night at Coast Camp, you can end your trip at the Point Reyes hostel by continuing 2.8 level miles on the Coast Trail, or at the Limantour Trailhead via 1.4 miles on the beach. Both of these options require a shuttle car. To make this a loop, return to the Sky Trailhead via the Fire Lane Trail, on a steep and exposed climb up the ridge.

BACKPACK Trip 6 | Glen and Wildcat camps from Bear Valley to Palomarin

SHUTTLE

First day: Bear Valley Trailhead to Glen Camp (4.6 miles)
Second day: Glen Camp to Wildcat Camp (2.7 miles)
Third day: Palomarin (5.7 miles)

After a level 3.1-mile walk on the Bear Valley Trail, you climb out of the creek canyon on the Glen Trail. Turn left on the Glen Camp Loop Trail in 0.6 mile to reach Glen Camp. The second day, ascend from the camp on the loop trail; pass the Greenpicker Trail and rejoin the Glen Trail 0.7 mile from the camp. Veer right on the Coast/Glen Spur South to reach the Coast Trail, and go left to descend the bluff above the ocean to the Stewart Trail. Turn left on the Stewart Trail to reach Wildcat Camp and Beach.

The next day, follow the Coast Trail for 5.7 undemanding miles to reach Palomarin.

Glen and Wildcat camps from Five Brooks

BACKPACK Trip 7

LOOP

First day: Five Brooks Trailhead to Glen Camp (4.9 miles)
Second day: Glen Camp to Wildcat Camp (2.7 miles)
Third day: Return to Five Brooks (6.4 miles on the Stewart Trail)

From the Five Brooks Trailhead, climb through dense forest on the Greenpicker Trail and then descend gently to the Glen Camp Loop Trail (4.4 miles from the trailhead). Turn right on the wide road to the camp, just a half mile downhill from the junction.

To reach the coast the next day, retrace your steps on the Glen Camp Loop Trail and then continue past the Greenpicker Trail for 0.2 mile to the Coast/Glen Spur South. Go left on the Coast Trail and descend the coastal bluff

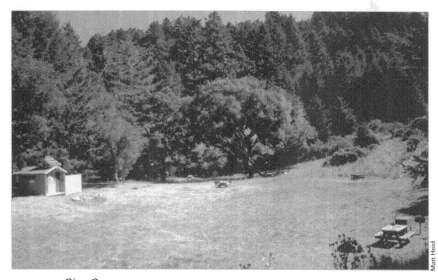

Glen Camp

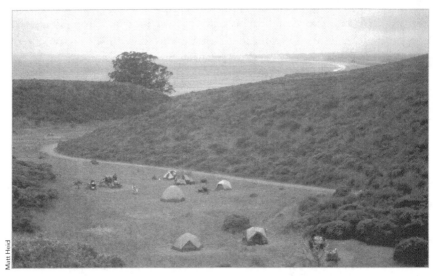

Coast Camp

(with views of Wildcat Lake and Double Point) to the Stewart Trail. Turn left for the final 0.7-mile downhill stretch to the camp.

After a night at Wildcat, you can return to Five Brooks any number of ways, the most straightforward being the Stewart Trail all the way. To avoid the steep climb to Firtop on the Stewart Trail, detour on the Ridge Trail.

Multi-day Trip

The Circuit

To really get away from it all, visit each campground in a four-night tour of the seashore.

First day: Sky Trailhead to Sky Camp, 1.3 miles
Second day: Sky Camp to Coast Camp, about 4 miles
Third day: Coast Camp to Glen Camp, 7.1 miles
Fourth day: Glen Camp to Wildcat Camp, 2.7 miles
Fifth day: Wildcat Camp to Palomarin, 5.7

Opposite page: Riding and Hiking Trail, Samuel P. Taylor State Park

Excursions in the Point Reyes Area

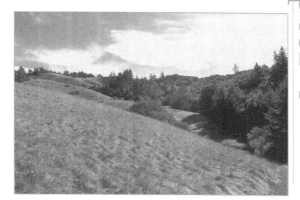

Chapter 6

TOMALES BAY STATE PARK

The bulk of Tomales Bay State Park lies on the west shore of the bay, protected from the Pacific's fog and wind by Inverness Ridge. Contoured bishop pines crown the ridge, and on its flanks, bay laurel, madrone, and oak join the pines; a luxuriant understory of coffeeberry, huckleberry, honeysuckle, sword fern, and salal (and abundant poison oak) flourishes in the fog-moistened soil.

Beachgoers will delight in the sheltered sandy coves; picnickers can choose between blufftop and beachside sites; hikers will find full-day hikes and short strolls through a rich forest to several beaches. On the east shore of Tomales Bay, a small parcel of the state park offers short walks along the beach and grassy bluff.

The west shore of Tomales Bay was once as enticing to developers as it is today to recreationists. The preservation of this land was the first challenge Bay Area conservationists undertook in the Point Reyes area: in 1945, reacting to the rapid acquisition of the bayshore by private owners, the Marin Conservation League bought 185 acres at Shell Beach for $30,000. This parcel and one that was purchased a few years later were turned over to the state of California in

1952 to become Tomales Bay State Park. The park is entirely surrounded by Point Reyes National Seashore except for a piece of land between Shell and Pebble beaches that remains in private hands today.

► WEST SHORE

See the map of Tomales Bay and Pierce Point Road areas on pages 166–167.

Driving Directions: From the Bear Valley Visitor Center, turn left on Bear Valley Road. Turn left again on Sir Francis Drake Highway, and continue through Inverness. Veer right on Pierce Point Road (2.5 miles beyond Inverness) and follow it a little over a mile to the signed entrance on the right.

After paying the entrance fee at the ranger station, follow the park road about a mile to parking and picnicking areas near Hearts Desire Beach.

Additional parking: About 350 yards south of the main entrance on Pierce Point Road, you can park in the roadside parking area and follow the Johnstone/Jepson Trail 0.7 mile to the picnic area at Hearts Desire Beach.

Facilities: At Hearts Desire Beach and picnic area: water, restrooms, dressing rooms, picnic tables, grills; boats may be carried from the parking lot and launched on the beach, away from swimming areas. Map available at ranger station. Campsites closed until further notice.

Hours: Every day from 8 A.M. to 8 P.M.

Regulations: Open during daylight hours; day use fee $4 per car, $3 for seniors 62 and over. Dogs allowed only in upper picnic area and must be leashed. No overnight parking.

Contact: (415) 669-1140; www.parks.ca.gov

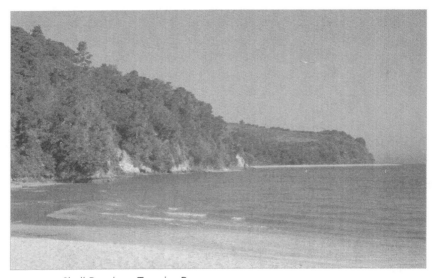

Shell Beach on Tomales Bay

WEST SHORE BEACHES

Unlike the beaches on the Pacific Coast, those on Tomales Bay are small, crescent-shaped coves, backed by rocky cliffs with thick, multi-layered vegetation. Alder branches hang low over the sand, and ceanothus, ocean spray, thimbleberry, and poison oak perch on the steep walls. Sticky monkeyflower, phacelia, and lizard tail brighten the cliffs when in bloom, and fleshy-leaved dudleya rosettes cling to the rocks. At low tide, you can walk a ways along the pebbly extensions of the beaches.

Swimmers will find the Tomales Bay waters less rough and less cold than Drakes Bay and the Pacific beaches. With Inverness Ridge buffering the wind and fog, the air is often warmer as well. However appealing the waters may be, note that there is no lifeguard service.

Regulations: None of the beaches in Tomales Bay State Park allow fires or camping

Shell Beach

Sunbathers and picnickers lounge on soft white sand, children play in the calm water, and swimmers are enticed by the floating raft anchored offshore in Tomales Bay. Shell Beach is a short walk from a parking area in residential Inverness.

Driving Directions: From the Bear Valley Visitor Center, turn left on Bear Valley Road. Turn left again on Sir Francis Drake Highway, and continue through Inverness to Camino del Mar (about a mile from the businesses) and turn right. The road ends at a small, shaded parking lot.

Facilities: Toilet at north end of Shell Beach I

The Beach: Two beaches actually comprise the singularly named Shell Beach— both are small, sheltered, and delightful. A smooth, 0.3-mile path, shaded by oak, bay laurel, and madrone, leads to the first beach from the parking lot. At the north end of Shell Beach I, a narrow path continues for 0.25 mile to Shell Beach II, where another delightful cove awaits. The beaches are separated from the rest of the park by a patch of private land. Hikers can reach Shell Beach from Hearts Desire Beach via a 4.3-mile trail that traverses the eastern slope of Inverness Ridge (or by a 2.8-mile trail from the parking pullout on Pierce Point Road).

Hearts Desire Beach

A great beach for picnics, wading, sand play, and kayak-launching.

Driving Directions: Access Hearts Desire from the main entrance road.

Facilities: Water, restrooms, dressing rooms, picnic tables, grills, kayak put-in, swimming

The Beach: On sunny weekends Hearts Desire Beach buzzes with activity. Families barbeque at beachside picnic spots, small children tote buckets and shovels to the shoreline, courageous souls test the water, and kayakers launch their crafts from the sandy bank. You're not likely to find much peace and quiet on weekends, but on weekdays you might have the beach to yourself. For a more secluded spot, take the nature trail to Indian Beach, just 0.4 mile to the north.

Indian Beach

This quiet beach is a long stretch of sand between Tomales Bay and a tidal marshland, just north of Hearts Desire Beach.

Facilities: Toilet, water

The Beach: You can reach Indian Beach on a 0.4-mile nature trail from Hearts Desire Beach (see Hiking Section). The blufftop path descends to the beach and crosses a wooden bridge over the marshy inlet from the bay. A reconstructed tepee on the beach recalls Coast Miwok settlements once present on Tomales Bay. The bay's rich marine life sustained Coast Miwok, who fished for salmon, herring, bass, and rock cod and foraged for clams and mussels.

Pebble Beach

Another scenic cove adjacent to Hearts Desire Beach.

Facilities: Toilet

The Beach: This broad cove, accessible via a 0.5-mile trail from Hearts Desire Beach, may be less busy on summer weekends than its neighbor. From Shell Beach, you can reach Pebble Beach on a 4.0-mile hike along the Johnstone Trail (see Hiking Section).

PICNICKING

You'll find picnic tables and grills in two locations at Hearts Desire Beach. At Vista Point, overlooking Tomales Bay, several tables beneath bishop pines on the bluff make a great gathering place for groups. Call the park to reserve (fee is $25 to $75, depending on the number of people). To reach the site by car, follow signs to the picnic area, veering right where beach-goers veer left into the beach parking lot. On foot, take the short path at the south end of Hearts Desire Beach.

For a picnic by the beach, you'll find several tables and grills in a grassy field just behind the sand, and beneath the shade of alder, big-leaf maple, and other riparian vegetation.

HIKING

Although small in size and traversed by few trails, Tomales Bay State Park offers a surprising number of options for hikers.

Nature Trail from Hearts Desire Beach to Indian Beach

A short nature trail leads from Hearts Desire Beach to Indian Beach (0.4 mile) and offers a loop possibility on the return. The path starts by the restrooms at Hearts Desire and climbs the hillside on a brief and gentle incline. Plaques along the way provide natural and cultural history information about blackberry, toyon, poison oak, and other plants that grow here, and how Coast Miwok used them.

After exploring Indian Beach, you can make a loop by walking a short way on the service road that begins by the toilet behind the beach. Veer left at a junction where the road branches right to Duck Cove and goes straight to Marshall Beach Road. You soon pick up the Nature Trail Loop and descend on a narrow path back to Indian Beach.

Pierce Point Road to Hearts Desire Beach

To combine a day at the beach with a short hike, you can leave your car at the roadside parking area on Pierce Point Road and follow the Jepson Trail downhill to Hearts Desire Beach. After 0.7 mile you reach the picnic area, and then continue a short way to the beach.

Hearts Desire Beach to Pebble Beach

A short excursion (0.5 mile) from Hearts Desire Beach takes you to neighboring Pebble Beach.

Jepson–Johnstone Loop

Trip 33

This short loop on the hillside above Tomales Bay offers a detour to Pebble Beach, a visit to the Jepson Memorial Grove of bishop pines, and fantastic views of the bay.

Distance: 2.6 miles
Type: Loop
Difficulty: Easy
Facilities: Water, restrooms, dressing rooms, picnic tables, grills, kayak put-in, swimming

Begin from the south end of Hearts Desire Beach. The trail climbs briefly to the blufftop picnic area and connects with the Johnstone Trail just beyond (named for Marin conservationist Bruce Johnstone). (A short detour leads to Pebble Beach.)

You ascend gradually beneath the shade of madrones, bishop pines, and large tanbark oaks. Coffeeberry, huckleberry, honeysuckle, and salal sprawl along the trail. After about a mile on the Johnstone Trail, you cross a paved road. (The road goes uphill about a quarter of a mile to the parking area on Pierce Point Road. Downhill, it leads to the parcel of land between Shell and Pebble beaches that is still privately owned.) Shortly beyond, you go right on the (signed) Jepson Trail. The trail climbs briefly, recrosses the road, and arrives at another junction where you continue straight, signed to HEARTS DESIRE BEACH. (Left goes to the parking area along Pierce Point Road.) Well-placed benches along the Jepson Trail offer spots to pause and take in the view through the trees of Tomales Bay. After a 0.7-mile gradual descent, you cross a paved road and reach the picnic-area parking lot. Pick up the trail on the other side and veer left through the picnic area to return to Hearts Desire Beach.

Jepson Grove

Once widespread along the California coast, bishop pines now grow only in scattered stands. Since the 1995 Vision Fire burned most of the pines on Inverness Ridge, the Jepson Memorial Grove in Tomales Bay State Park is one of the few remaining virgin bishop-pine forests. The grove is named for Willis Linn Jepson, author of the monumental classic, *Manual of the Flowering Plants of California*.

Hearts Desire Beach to Shell Beach

Talk a walk through the rich forest on the slopes of Inverness Ridge, with views of the bay as you go and a beach at your starting and finishing points. Ideally, you'll find a friend who would rather spend a day a the beach than hike, and who is willing to shuttle you the short distance between these trailheads. If not, you can easily leave a car at the Shell Beach parking area and continue to Hearts Desire to begin your hike. For a full-day excursion, with some beach time at both ends, make this an out-and-back hike. If you begin from the parking area along Pierce Point Road, you'll shorten this hike by about a mile and a half. However, you'll miss Hearts Desire Beach.

Distance: 4.6 miles one-way
Type: Shuttle
Difficulty: Moderate
Facilities: Water, restrooms, dressing rooms, picnic tables, grills, kayak put-in, swimming

Begin from the south end of Hearts Desire Beach on the path to the blufftop picnic area. After a brief climb, the path passes through a grassy area with tables

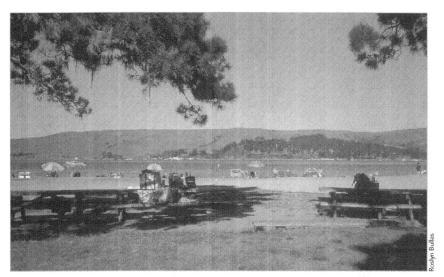

Hearts Desire Beach

and connects with the Johnstone Trail just beyond (named for Marin conservationist Bruce Johnstone).

You ascend gradually beneath the shade of madrones, bishop pines, and large tanbark oaks. For most of this route, coffeeberry, huckleberry, honeysuckle, and salal sprawl along the trail. After about a mile on the Johnstone Trail, you cross a paved road. (The road goes uphill about a quarter of a mile to the parking area on Pierce Point Road. Downhill, it leads to the parcel of land between Shell and Pebble beaches that is still privately owned.) Shortly beyond, you reach a junction with the Jepson Trail and continue straight on the Johnstone Trail, signed SHELL BEACH. After a gentle, switchbacking climb, you contour at about 500 feet on the hillside above Tomales Bay, where occasional grassy patches and breaks in the forest allow views across the water. After a couple of miles, the trail begins to descend gradually through tanbark oak and madrone, and after several switchbacks emerges at the north end of Shell Beach II. To find your car, continue across the beach to the short trail to Shell Beach I, cross that beach, and pick up the 0.3-mile path to the parking lot.

► EAST SHORE BEACH
Millerton Point and Alan Sieroty Beach
A bayside beach and a grassy mesa with spring wildflowers provide short walks with great views of the surrounding bay and highlands. Look for osprey in the nest on top of an unused utility pole.

Driving Directions: Go north on Highway 1 from Point Reyes Station for 4.5 miles. Turn left into the parking area, marked by several large eucalyptus trees.

Facilities: Toilet, picnic tables
Regulations: Dogs on leash, no bikes, no horses
Contact: (415) 669-1140; www.parks.ca.gov
The Beach: A narrow stretch of beach borders this point of land that juts into Tomales Bay. Follow the left-hand path, which leaves the parking area to quickly arrive at the beach. You can follow the pebbly sand all the way around the point and then head back to the parking lot on small paths across the grassy bluff.

Along the edge of the blufftop, an old farm road provides views of offshore oyster beds in Tomales Bay.

Osprey Outpost

A platform atop a lone utility pole on the bluff at Millerton Point holds an osprey nest. The osprey originally built their nest on a wired power pole, but after it caused a short in power to Inverness, PG&E constructed a pole just for the birds, and successfully encouraged the ospreys to move their home. You can often see adult birds flying to and from the nest, feeding their chicks.

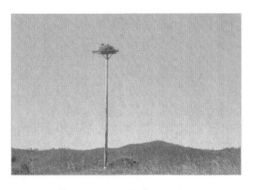

Osprey nest at Millerton Point

During the 1960s, pesticide contamination in rivers severely reduced populations of fish-eating birds like osprey. Researchers determined that DDT and related pesticides were the most harmful to the birds; after DDT was banned in 1972, osprey populations began to expand again. Today, there are about 20 nests on Inverness Ridge, and the birds soar above Tomales Bay and Bolinas Lagoon, searching for fish in the waters below.

GOLDEN GATE NATIONAL RECREATION AREA

The world's largest urban national park, the Golden Gate National Recreation Area encompasses 75,398 acres and 28 miles of coastline in the San Francisco Bay Area. From pockets of parkland along the perimeter of San Francisco, like Ocean Beach and Crissy Field, to miles of trails in open space at the Marin Headlands and Bolinas Ridge, the GGNRA offers diverse and unique experiences. Around Point Reyes, GGNRA land includes Bolinas Ridge, the east side of the Olema Valley, and a small holding along Tomales Bay, all managed by Point Reyes National Seashore.

Facilities: No toilets or water on the GGNRA trails in this book.
Regulations: Dogs on leash
Contact: Point Reyes National Seashore manages the area of the GGNRA included in this book. Contact the Bear Valley Visitor Center for information regarding these trails. (415) 464-5100

Bolinas Ridge Trail

The Bolinas Ridge Trail begins on the pastoral ridgeline east of Olema Valley. Especially popular with mountain bikers, the trail crosses rolling coastal rangeland, enters towering redwoods, and breaks into open chaparral before it reaches its southern trailhead at Alpine Road on Mt. Tamalpais. You'll enjoy far-reaching views of Bolinas Lagoon, Tomales Bay, and the Pacific Ocean. In sunny Olema Valley, this trip is a good choice when fog blankets the coast.

Distance: Up to 11.1 miles one-way
Type: Out-and-back or shuttle
Difficulty: Easy to strenuous
Facilities: None
Regulations: Bikes and dogs allowed
Driving Directions: From Hwy. 101, take Sir Francis Drake Blvd. 19.3 miles to the trailhead at the crest of the hill on the south side of the road. From Point Reyes National Seashore headquarters at Bear Valley, turn right on Bear Valley Road, and right again on Highway 1. Make a left on Sir Francis Drake Highway at the stop sign. Follow it to the crest of the hill, where you'll see a cattle stile and a trail heading over the grasslands. Park along the road.

For a shuttle hike, or to begin at the other end, from Hwy. 101, take Sir Francis Drake Blvd. 5.3 miles to Pacheco Dr. in Fairfax and

Trip 35

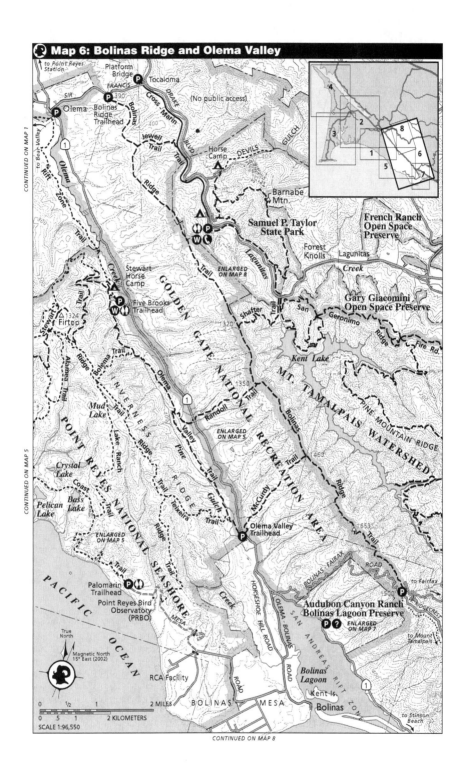

to Point Reyes Station
Platform Bridge
Tocaloma
FRANCIS
SIR
(No public access)
Olema
Bolinas Ridge Trailhead
DRAKE
Cross Marin
BLVD.
390
Jewell Trail
Bolinas
Horse Camp
DEVILS
GULCH
400
CONTINUED ON MAP 1
to Bear Valley
SIR
Olema
Rift
Zone
Trail
300
Ridge
Trail
Barnabe Mtn.
Samuel P. Taylor State Park
French Ranch Open Space Preserve
ENLARGED ON MAP 8
Forest Knolls
Lagunitas
Lagunitas
Creek
Stewart Horse Camp
GOLDEN
Trail
Lagunitas
Shafter
Trail
San
Gary Giacomini Open Space Preserve
Geronimo
Ridge
Fire Rd.
Creek
Five Brooks Trailhead
1324
Firtop
GATE
1320
Kent Lake
MT.
TAMALPAIS
Stewart
Ridge
Bolema
Trail
Alamere
Trail
NATIONAL
1350
Olema
Valley
Trail
Randall
Trail
Bolinas
WATERSHED
PINE
MOUNTAIN
RIDGE
CONTINUED ON MAP 5
Mud Lake
INVERNESS
Lake
Ranch
Trail
RECREATION
1
Trail
1460
Ridge
POINT
Crystal Lake
Coast
Trail
RIDGE
Pine
Gulch
Trail
McCurdy
Trail
AREA
Pelican Lake
Bass Lake
Teixeira
Trail
Olema Valley Trailhead
1653
Trail
200
REYES
ENLARGED ON MAP 5
Ridge
Trail
Trail
Creek
BOLINAS-FAIRAX
ROAD
to Fairfax
NATIONAL
Palomarin Trailhead
Trail
MESA
HORSESHOE HILL ROAD
OLEMA-BOLINAS
1500
Audubon Canyon Ranch Bolinas Lagoon Preserve
ENLARGED ON MAP 7
to Mount Tamalpais
SEASHORE
Point Reyes Bird Observatory (PRBO)
SAN
ANDREAS
RIFT
ZONE
PACIFIC
True North
Magnetic North 15° East (2002)
RCA Facility
ROAD
ROAD
Bolinas Lagoon
Kent Is.
1
OCEAN
BOLINAS
MESA
Bolinas
to Stinson Beach
0   ½   1   2 MILES
0 .5 1   2 KILOMETERS
SCALE 1:96,550

CONTINUED ON MAP 8

turn left (west). Turn right on Broadway and then left onto Bolinas Rd. Continue past Alpine Dam (at 7.5 miles) to Ridgecrest Blvd. (9.0 miles). Park on the side of the road. The trail begins just north of the junction.

Squeeze through the wooden cattle guard and follow the narrow path that quickly meets the main route. On a gentle incline, the wide trail climbs through cow-grazed grasslands, passing gullies where bay laurel and Douglas-fir trees grow in thick clumps. During the summer and fall, these vibrant evergreen trees contrast with golden grassy slopes; in spring, glossy yellow buttercups dot green pastures. After 1 mile you reach the first of many cattle gates and stiles you'll pass through on this route. You meet the Jewell Trail at 1.3 miles, which descends the eastern slope to reach the Cross Marin Trail through Samuel P. Taylor State Park.

The trail grows wilder as it continues, and fewer cows graze the hillsides (although you'll go through a number of cattle gates or stiles along this stretch of the trail). Occasional brief climbs offset stretches of fairly level and exposed trail, lined with coyote bush and blackberry. Small, reed-rimmed ponds occupy low depressions, and Douglas-fir, oak, and bay laurel grow where the hills ripple together.

View from the Trail

The Bolinas Ridge Trail affords fantastic views: the folds of volcanic Black Mountain, the high peak of Barnabe Mountain, the elongated finger of Tomales Bay, and the low trough of the Olema Valley. The San Andreas fault runs the length of the bay and valley, and its movement formed the bay and Bolinas Lagoon at the other end of the valley. From Bolinas Ridge, you have a great perspective on the mismatched hills that rise from the valley on opposite sides of the fault, indicating its presence: low, rolling grasslands to the east, and a high, thickly vegetated ridge to the west.

The open pastures begin to give way to an increasingly dense forest, and you climb steadily, passing junctions with the Shafter Trail (5.2 miles), the Randall Trail (6.1 miles), and the McCurdy Trail (7.7 miles). Towering coast redwoods and Douglas-firs envelop the wide, duff-covered trail, with ferns and evergreen huckleberry, and springtime Douglas iris and milkmaids in the understory. As you continue, occasional breaks in the trees yield views of Bolinas Lagoon and the Pacific to the west, through tall bushes of manzanita. To the east, Pine Mountain Ridge rises above rolling hills.

You soon emerge in open chaparral on a hard-packed dirt and rocky surface. Manzanita, ceanothus, and scrub oak shield the coast from view. The trail rolls up and down, but mostly up, as you approach the southern end of the trail.

The Bolinas Ridge Trail is one link in the Bay Area Ridge Trail—a 400+-mile route that will eventually encircle the entire bay. To continue on the Bay Area Ridge Trail route, descend the Jewell Trail (which begins 1.3 miles from the trailhead on Sir Francis Drake Highway), where you'll have great views of Black Mountain. In 0.9-mile you reach the Cross Marin Trail in Samuel P. Taylor State Park (see page 230), where you can go left and continue 1.5 level miles on a paved trail to Platform Bridge on Sir Francis Drake Highway. (Roadside parking available for shuttle car.) Or turn left on the Cross Marin Trail and follow the paved trail 2.1 miles to Samuel P. Taylor Park Headquarters. The Bay Area Ridge Trail will eventually traverse the park to reach the next segment on Mt. Burdell in Novato.

The Shafter Trail, which descends from the Bolinas Ridge Trail after 5.2 miles from the trailhead, is closed between December and June to protect spawning coho salmon in Lagunitas Creek. In summer and fall, you can make a loop on the Shafter, Bolinas Ridge, Jewell, and Cross Marin trails.

Trip 36

Bolinas Ridge and Olema Valley Loop

The Randall and McCurdy trails link the upper reaches of Bolinas Ridge with the Olema Valley Trail. This trip gives you a taste of the variety of landscapes you can visit in just a few hours—dense redwood and Douglas-fir forest, pastoral grasslands, peaceful meadows, and fragrant chaparral—all rewards for a steep climb on the Randall Trail and an even steeper descent on the McCurdy Trail. **Note:** You might encounter some boggy patches on the Olema Valley Trail during wet months, and a creek crossing shortly beyond the trailhead might require you to take off your shoes.

Distance: 8 miles
Difficulty: Strenuous
Type: Loop
Facilities: None
Regulations: No dogs or bikes on Olema Valley Trail; dogs and bikes allowed on Randall, McCurdy, and Bolinas Ridge trails (in GGNRA)
Driving Directions: From Olema, go south on Highway 1 for 8 miles to the signed OLEMA VALLEY TRAILHEAD on the west side of the highway. Park along the road.

A 0.4-mile connector path leads from the trailhead to a junction with the Olema Valley and Teixeira trails. Wade through the high grasses toward the forested slope that rises from the valley floor. You soon reach a creek crossing, which may require you to take off your shoes in wet months, and shortly after the crossing you arrive at the junction. Veer right on the Olema Valley Trail and begin your trip up the valley along the San Andreas fault, through grasslands and oak and bay forests.

After 2.4 miles on the Olema Valley Trail, you reach a spur trail to the Randall Trailhead on Highway 1. Turn right and in 0.4 mile cross the highway to pick up the trail on the other side. On warm days, several cars are often parked in the roadside pullout at the trailhead, some belonging to bathers at Hagmaier Pond, a swimming hole near the old Randall ranchhouse.

The wide Randall Trail, an old ranch road, climbs steeply through a shady Douglas-fir forest and reaches the Bolinas Ridge Trail in 1.7 miles from Highway 1. The Ridge Trail meanders gently uphill (southeast) for another 1.6 miles, shaded by tall redwoods. Tanbark oak grows in the understory, and springtime milkmaids and iris enliven the forest. Turn left on the McCurdy Trail, which quickly descends from the trees to become a steep, rutted route back into Olema Valley. Views of Stinson Beach peek through tall bushes of fragrant chaparral. You pass through a stretch of Douglas-fir and tanbark oak that shade the trail, and then emerge on an open hillside above the valley. The trail becomes a narrow path over grasslands, in spring decorated with blue-eyed grass and buttercups. After 1.9 miles from the Ridge Trail you reach the trailhead at Highway 1.

Tomales Bay Trail

Trip 37

This short walk crosses pastures to reach two small ponds with lots of birdlife. Continue to the low bluffs above Tomales Bay, where you'll have terrific views of the surrounding area.

Distance: 2.6 miles
Type: Out-and-back
Difficulty: Easy
Facilities: None
Regulations: No dogs, horses, bikes, or camping
Driving Directions: Go north on Highway 1 for 1.5 miles from Point Reyes Station. Turn left into the gravel parking lot.

Follow the small path across the grasslands and past an interesting rock outcropping. The trail widens as it descends to two small ponds, flanked by willows, coyote bush, and poison oak. Ducks, red-winged blackbirds, and other birds

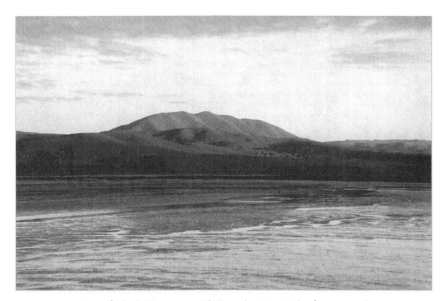
A view of Black Mountain with Tomales Bay in the foreground

gather near the water. Beyond the ponds, you ascend a slight rise, and top out on a low hillside above Tomales Bay.

You have expansive views from the shore above Tomales Bay marshlands: as you stand on the North American Plate, you're looking across the San Andreas fault to the Pacific Plate. The bare trunks of trees burned in the 1995 Vision Fire are still prominent on Inverness Ridge. Look north along the peninsula as it stretches to the mouth of Tomales Bay at Tomales Point. East and southeast, Black and Barnabe mountains rise from rolling inland hills. Retrace your steps to the trailhead.

AUDUBON CANYON RANCH BOLINAS LAGOON PRESERVE

More than 100 pairs of great blue herons and great and snowy egrets nest in the lofty branches of redwood trees at the Bolinas Lagoon Preserve. Herons and egrets returned each spring to this grove of redwoods on the slopes of Bolinas Ridge long before the dairy ranch on this site became the 1000-acre Audubon Canyon Ranch preserve.

On a short trail from the picnic area and visitor center, you reach an overlook where powerful viewing scopes look directly into the nests. In March and early April, you'll see courting rituals and nest-building. Bright eggs appear in the nests by April and May, and a few tiny heads of newborn chicks. Visit in June and July to see the chicks noisily demanding food from their parents, who make foraging missions to Bolinas Lagoon, Tomales Bay, and beyond.

The picnic area in Picher Canyon offers a great view of the egrets and herons near the tops of the tall redwoods. Visit the display hall to learn about the history of the preserve and the natural history of the area. The bookstore next door offers a great selection of maps, guides, and other interesting reading.

Driving Directions: From Highway 101, north or south, take the Sir Francis Drake exit and head west for about 21 miles to reach the town of Olema. Turn left (south) on Highway 1 and continue for about 11 miles to Audubon Canyon Ranch, on the left side of the highway, opposite Bolinas Lagoon.

To approach Audubon Canyon Ranch from the south on Highway 1, take the Highway 1/Stinson Beach exit from Highway 101. Follow Highway 1 for about 12 miles to Stinson Beach. Go through town and continue for about 3 miles, past Volunteer Canyon, to the main preserve entrance, on the right side of the highway.

Facilities: Water, restrooms, phone, picnic tables, bookstore, and exhibit hall. All facilities, a teaching pond, and a viewing area in the ranch yard are wheelchair-accessible; trails and overlook are not.

Regulations: No fee, but donations welcomed; no dogs; no smoking

Hours: Open weekends and holidays from 10 A.M. to 4 P.M., from the second weekend in March through the second weekend in July. Schools and other groups can make appointments Tuesdays through Fridays.

Contact: (415) 868-9244; www.egret.org

HENDERSON OVERLOOK

A scenic half-mile trail leads to the preserve's main attraction—the Henderson Overlook. A small path signed to the overlook leaves the entrance road and climbs briefly up the hillside through a lush coat of hazelnut, coffeeberry, tanbark oak, and ceanothus, with iris in prolific bloom beneath. You quickly reach a small plateau with a view over Bolinas Lagoon. Low tide reveals a mosaic of

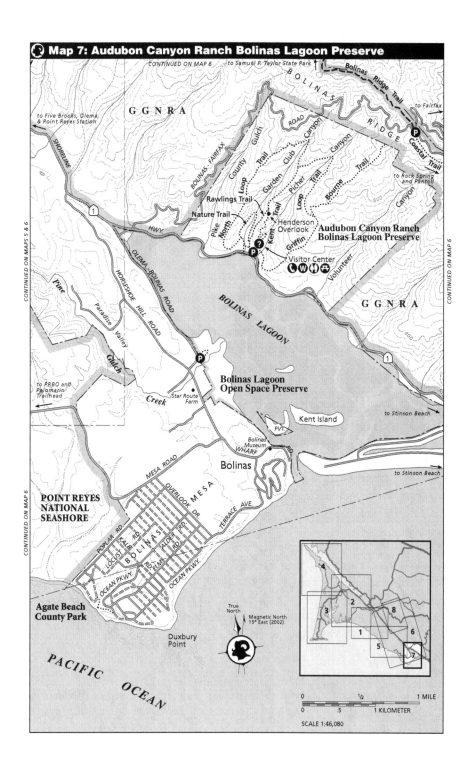

Map 7: Audubon Canyon Ranch Bolinas Lagoon Preserve

CONTINUED ON MAP 6

to Samuel P. Taylor State Park

Bolinas Ridge Trail

BOLINAS RIDGE

to Fairfax

GGNRA

to Five Brooks, Olema, & Point Reyes Station

SHORELINE

BOLINAS-FAIRFAX ROAD

Gulch

County Loop Trail

Canyon

Garden Club Trail

Picher Canyon

Bourne Trail

to Rock Spring and Pantoll

Canyon

Rawlings Trail

Nature Trail

Pike

North

Loop

Trail

Kent Trail

Henderson Overlook

Griffin

Audubon Canyon Ranch Bolinas Lagoon Preserve

Volunteer

Visitor Center

GGNRA

CONTINUED ON MAPS 5 & 6

CONTINUED ON MAP 6

HWY 1

OLEMA-BOLINAS ROAD

HORSESHOE HILL ROAD

Pine

Paradise Valley

Gulch

to PRBO and Palomarin Trailhead

Creek

BOLINAS LAGOON

Star Route Farm

Bolinas Lagoon Open Space Preserve

Kent Island

to Stinson Beach

Bolinas Museum

WHARF

PVT.

RD.

to Stinson Beach

Bolinas

POINT REYES NATIONAL SEASHORE

MESA ROAD

OVERLOOK DR.

MESA

TERRACE AVE.

POPLAR RD.

KALE RD.

LOCUST RD.

BOLINAS

ELM RD.

ALDER RD.

OCEAN PKWY.

OCEAN PKWY.

Agate Beach County Park

Duxbury Point

True North

Magnetic North 15° East (2002)

PACIFIC OCEAN

4

2

3

8

1

6

5

7

0 — 1/2 — 1 MILE

0 — .5 — 1 KILOMETER

SCALE 1:46,080

narrow water channels. Spotting scopes provide a closer look at the herons, egrets, sandpipers, pelicans, osprey, and other bird species that feed in the mud-flats. Large colonies of harbor seals haul out on the flats at low tide.

Continue climbing through a dense forest of lush spring growth. The trail soon levels and a small sign in the bushes asks you to be quiet because you are approaching the overlook. A short spur dips down to the viewing spot, where wooden benches provide a spot to rest and to contemplate the birds from afar, and several spotting scopes offer an up-close view of the nests. A knowledgeable volunteer is always stationed at the overlook.

You can return on a short trail that descends directly to the picnic area and offers another spot to view the birds through telescopes, or explore the other trails that loop through the preserve.

BIRDS OF THE BOLINAS LAGOON PRESERVE

Herons arrive at the preserve toward the end of January, followed by egrets in mid-March. Soon after they arrive, the birds begin courtship rituals, displaying long feather plumes and presenting twigs to their mates. Each female lays between two and five eggs, and incubation lasts about 28 days. Once the eggs have hatched, adults leave the nest to make regular foraging missions for the hungry chicks, who squabble noisily over food when their parents return.

Young egrets first test their wings at about seven weeks of age, and herons wait until nine weeks. If you visit in June or July, you may be lucky enough to see a first flight.

LOOP TRAILS

Once you've seen the egrets and herons, visit the preserve's varied habitats on two loop trails. You might glimpse some of the more than 90 species of land-birds that live here, and perhaps a brush rabbit, gray fox, or bobcat as well.

Both loops are about 3 miles and begin from the overlook. Return to the main trail and continue uphill through the redwood, Douglas-fir, and bay laurel forest. After a steady climb, the trail forks: the **Griffin Loop** goes right and circles Picher Canyon; **Zumie's Loop** branches left and descends the fern-covered slopes of Garden Club Canyon Creek. Both trails offer a combination of quiet forest, sun-dappled meadow, and open chaparral, and provide views of Bolinas Lagoon.

The three-quarter-mile **self-guided nature trail** loop offers an easy and educational stroll. You can pick up a map and a guide in the bookstore or from one of the hosts who greeted you as you came in.

HISTORY OF THE PRESERVE

The redwoods on Bolinas Ridge were once home to one of the largest populations of great blue herons on the West Coast of the United States. In fact, great numbers of herons nested throughout the San Francisco Bay Area until logging and urbanization destroyed most of their habitat. The timber frenzy of the mid-1800s felled most old-growth trees, and urbanization encroached on nesting and feeding sites.

When the Bay Area's population surged after World War II, Marin County made elaborate plans to develop the coast, and the heronry at Bolinas Lagoon was in imminent danger: the dairy ranch that occupied the present-day preserve site was slated to be logged and subdivided, Bolinas Lagoon would be dredged and a marina built, and a four-lane highway along the coast would separate the birds' nesting site and feeding grounds—likely the final blow to the birds, which depended on the redwoods and the nearby tidelands.

In the early 1960s, members of the Marin Audubon Society began a fundraising campaign that ultimately succeeded in purchasing the large swath of land that is today Audubon Canyon Ranch.

OTHER AUDUBON CANYON RANCH PRESERVES

Although the Bolinas Lagoon Preserve is the only Audubon Canyon Ranch holding open to the public in the Point Reyes area, ACR owns and manages almost 500 acres in 12 sites around Tomales Bay. The Cypress Grove Research Center, on the east shore of the bay, is ACR's research headquarters. The immediate access to the bay environment provides staff at the preserve with an ideal opportunity to study shorebirds and waterbirds and their habitats.

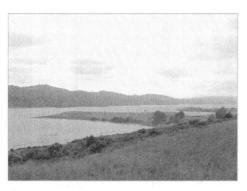

Tomales Bay, east shore

The quaint Victorian buildings at Cypress Grove were originally built as a whistlestop for the farm up the hill when the North Pacific Coast Railroad routed its line along Tomales Bay. In the 1950s, Clifford Conly purchased the land, and bit by bit began donating it to ACR. Cypress Grove is open to the public only during special events, workshops, and seminars.

ACR also runs the Bouverie Preserve in Sonoma. You can visit the preserve by making an appointment, by signing up for one of the guided nature walks, or by joining a work-day event to help clear trails and plant in the gardens.

SAMUEL P. TAYLOR STATE PARK

Redwoods don't grow at Point Reyes, because of the peninsula's unique geology, but you don't have to go far to find them. Just a few miles from Point Reyes, east of the San Andreas fault, Samuel P. Taylor State Park is a redwood haven. The impressive giants tower above Lagunitas Creek, which runs through the park, and shade the park's campgrounds and picnic areas.

But Samuel P. Taylor offers much more than redwoods. Tucked in the rolling hills of West Marin, the park encompasses 2800 acres of grasslands, mixed oak and bay laurel forests, and creekside redwoods. Coho salmon and steelhead trout spawn in several tributaries of Lagunitas Creek that run through the park.

To the east, the forested slope of Bolinas Ridge often protects the park from coastal weather patterns; when fog hangs near the coast, you're likely to find sun baking these grassy hills, but on hot days, the deep redwood forests offer a cool refuge.

Hikers, bicyclists, and equestrians will find narrow paths, fire roads, and nature trails that traverse the park along Devils Gulch and Lagunitas (Papermill) creeks and up to Barnabe Mountain. You can choose from level, moderate, or steep routes.

Driving Directions: From Hwy. 101 take Sir Francis Drake Blvd. for 15 miles to the main park entrance and campground, on the right.

Facilities: Water, restrooms, phone, picnic tables, campsites; trail map available for $1

Regulations: Day use fee $4 per car

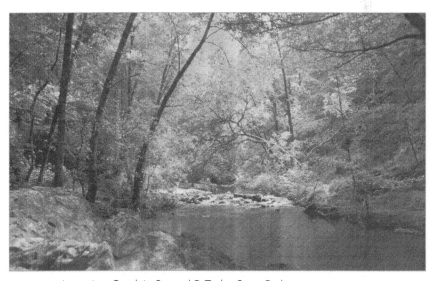

Lagunitas Creek in Samuel P. Taylor State Park

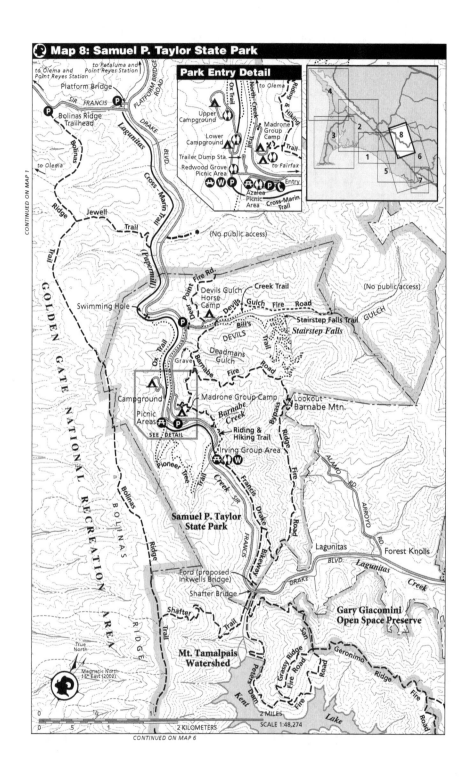

Park Entry Detail

to Petaluma and Point Reyes Station

to Olema and Point Reyes Station

Platform Bridge

SIR FRANCIS

Bolinas Ridge Trailhead

to Olema

Ox Trail

to Olema

Upper Campground

North Creek Trail

Riding & Hiking

Madrone Group Camp

Lower Campground

Trailer Dump Sta.

Trail

Redwood Grove Picnic Area

to Fairfax

Entry

Azalea Picnic Area

Cross-Marin Trail

Jewell

Trail

(No public access)

Devils Gulch Horse Camp

Creek Trail

Devils Gulch Fire Road

(No public access)

Swimming Hole

Bill's

Stairstep Falls Trail

GULCH

Stairstep Falls

DEVILS

Deadmans Gulch

Trail

Gravel

Barnabe

Fire

Road

Campground

Madrone Group Camp

Lookout Barnabe Mtn.

Picnic Areas

Barnabe Creek

Bypass

SEE DETAIL

Riding & Hiking Trail

Irving Group Area

Pioneer Tree Trail

Creek

Francis

Drake

Bikeway

SIR FRANCIS

Ridge Fire Road

ALAMO RD.

ARROYO

RD.

Samuel P. Taylor State Park

Lagunitas

Forest Knolls

BLVD.

Lagunitas

Ford (proposed Inkwells Bridge)

DRAKE

Creek

Shafter Bridge

Gary Giacomini Open Space Preserve

Shafter Trail

True North

Mt. Tamalpais Watershed

Peters Dam

Grassy Ridge Fire Road

Geronimo

Ridge

Fire

Road

Magnetic North 15° East (2002)

Kent

Lake

0   1/2   1

0   .5   1

2 KILOMETERS

2 MILES

SCALE 1:48,274

GOLDEN GATE NATIONAL RECREATION AREA

BOLINAS RIDGE

Lagunitas (Papermill)

Cross-Marin Trail

Bolinas Ridge

PLATFORM BRIDGE ROAD

DRAKE BLVD.

Point Fire Rd.

Deer Trail

Ox Trail

CONTINUED ON MAP 1

CONTINUED ON MAP 6

Dogs allowed only in campground and paved areas and must be on a 6-foot (maximum) leash.

Bikes allowed on fire roads, on paved Cross Marin Trail, and in campground and picnic areas. Must observe 15 MPH speed limit on fire roads and 5 MPH on curves. Helmet required.

Horses allowed on fire roads and the Ox and Pioneer Tree trails

Contact: (415) 488-9897; www.parks.ca.gov

CAMPING

Sixty-one family campsites border Lagunitas Creek beneath towering redwoods in Samuel P. Taylor State Park. Each site has a picnic table, fire ring, food locker, and parking space. Drinking water and restrooms with hot showers are located nearby. There are no electricity, water, or sewage hook-ups for trailers. You can purchase firewood at the ranger station. Up to eight people are allowed in each campsite, with a maximum of two vehicles.

There is one shared campsite that accommodates bicyclists and hikers who are passing through the park. Campsites cost $15 per night between May 15 and September 15 and $12 the rest of the year.

Devils Gulch Horse Camp, 1 mile west of the main park entrance and campground, has one campsite for equestrians only, which accommodates up to 20 people, 12 horses, and six vehicles ($15 per night includes two horses; $2 for each additional horse); two group campsites at Devils Gulch are open to non-equestrian groups of up to 10 people and three vehicles ($14 per night). **Madrone Group Campground**, a quarter-mile west of the main entrance, has two group sites that accommodate 50 people ($67 per night) and 25 people ($34).

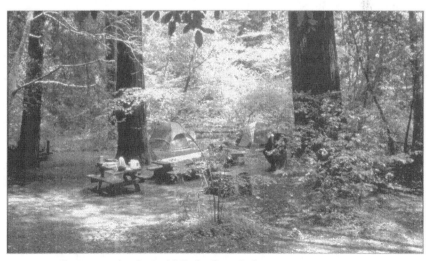

Campground at Samuel P. Taylor State Park

Reserve America handles all campsite reservations in Samuel P. Taylor State Park. Call (800) 444-7275 up to seven months in advance. During peak season, the campground usually fills right away, so plan your trip early.

PICNICKING

All picnic areas provide tables, grills, water, and toilets. Near the campground at the main entrance, the **Azalea Picnic Area** is next to the creek, shaded by redwoods. You cannot reserve in advance, so be sure to arrive early, especially on weekends and holidays. The area opens at 8 A.M. every day; closing time varies according to season.

Across the creek, the **Redwood Group Picnic Area** accommodates up to 80 people and 30 vehicles ($90 per day). The **Irving Group Picnic Area**, 1 mile east of the main entrance on Sir Francis Drake Highway, accommodates up to 30 people and 15 vehicles ($45 per day). Make reservations for both group sites through Reserve America at (800) 444-7275.

Papermill to State Park

Samuel Penfield Taylor arrived in California in 1850, one of thousands who sought their fortune in the gold rush. Unlike most 49ers, Taylor found gold, and he used his earnings to buy 100 acres of prime redwood forest along Lagunitas Creek. He built a successful papermill that supplied San Francisco newspapers and businesses with newsprint and fine paper. In 1874, the North Pacific Coast Railroad was routed through the creek canyon on its way to Point Reyes, making the previously isolated area easily reachable from the big city. Taylor turned his land beneath the redwoods along Lagunitas Creek into a resort area, and Camp Taylor became one of the most popular weekend recreation areas in California, and one of the first places in the United States where people went for outdoor camping.

SALMON—VIEWING SPOTS

Coho salmon were once bountiful in West Marin creeks; historic accounts report virtual silver rivers of salmon—3000 to 5000 fish annually. Over the past century, dams, logging, road construction, fires, and gravel mining have all contributed to the destruction of salmon habitat in the Lagunitas Creek watershed. The number of fish in Lagunitas Creek decreased dramatically in the 1940s, and coho salmon are now federally listed as a threatened species. Local groups have begun to work on creek restoration to recover salmon habitat, and the Marin Municipal Water District is conducting a long-term restoration project to reduce sediments in the creeks and improve conditions for migrating salmon. (See pagess 36–38 for more information about the life cycle of coho salmon and the Point Reyes National Seashore restoration program.)

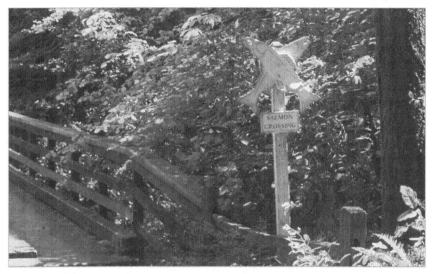

Salmon sign

The best months to look for spawning coho salmon in West Marin creeks are December and January, especially a couple days after a big rainstorm. You have a good chance of seeing the fish from three sites in and around Samuel P. Taylor State Park. At the **main park entrance**, a small path near the ranger station leads to the creek bank, and interpretive plaques nearby tell you about salmon habitat and life cycle.

A path along the creek at **Devils Gulch** provides excellent salmon-viewing points and a peaceful stroll through the riparian forest. From the Devils Gulch trailhead (see Trip 46), walk up the paved road 0.1 mile to a narrow path that branches right and follows the creek. Pass the bridge and continue on the left side of the creek for about 1 mile, until the path ends at a gate.

Shafter Bridge is a convenient road-side spot where you have a good chance of seeing salmon from the bank above Lagunitas Creek. The bridge is on Sir Francis Drake Highway about 2 miles east of the main park entrance and a half mile west of the town of Lagunitas. Marin Municipal Water District opens the parking area next to the bridge between December and mid-February. Call (415) 459-5267 for more information.

Salmon Watching

You're most likely to see salmon if they don't see you. Stay on the banks of the creek, away from the water. Don't throw anything into the creek, and be sure your footing doesn't cause rocks or soil to slide into the water. Disturbing salmon habitat is harmful to the fish and reduces your chances of seeing salmon spawning and resting.

Note: The distances on state park signs are given first in kilometers, with miles in parentheses.

Trip 38 | Cross Marin Trail

Distance: 3.5 miles one-way
Type: Out-and-back
Difficulty: Easy
Regulations: Bikes, horses, and leashed dogs allowed

The paved Cross Marin Trail that snakes through Samuel P. Taylor State Park is a level, creekside route, perfect for a family bike outing. From the campground at the main park entrance to the Platform Bridge in Tocaloma, the paved trail follows the route of the North Pacific Coast Railroad that ran from Sausalito to Cazadero, in the heart of the North Coast timber country.

Trip 39 | Pioneer Nature Trail

Distance: 2.2-mile
Type: Loop
Difficulty: Easy
Regulations: No bikes or dogs; horses allowed

A pamphlet available at the ranger station tells you about the plants and animals on this short interpretive trail. To reach the trail from the ranger station, follow the road across the bridge over Lagunitas Creek and go left to the Redwood Group Picnic Area (parking available here). Just beyond the fire-road gate, pick up the Pioneer Trail where it begins to climb gently along Wildcat Creek. The trail winds through the redwood forest, flanked by tanbark oak, hazelnut, and ferns. Look for the interpretive signposts about redwoods, fire, the pioneer tree, and forest ecology in the guide. Watch for poison oak.

You soon begin to descend alongside another creek and then reach the Cross Marin Trail. Go left and return to the campground in 0.6 mile.

Stairstep Falls

This scenic walk is great anytime of year, but it is especially beautiful in late fall and winter, when big-leaf maple leaves turn the forest into a tapestry of red and gold, salmon spawn in the creek, and Stairstep Falls gushes with water.

Distance: 2.8 miles
Type: Out-and-back
Difficulty: Easy
Facilities: Toilets, water, picnic tables, and grills at Devils Gulch Horse Camp
Regulations: No dogs on trail
Driving Directions: Continue on Sir Francis Drake Highway for 1 mile beyond the main park entrance and campground to the signed DEVILS GULCH HORSE CAMP on the right side of the road. Park in the gravel pullout on the left.

Follow the paved road from Sir Francis Drake Highway beneath the cover of bay laurel, big-leaf maple, California buckeye, and alder that grow in the riparian canyon of Devils Gulch Creek. After 0.1 mile, a narrow dirt path branches right and approaches the creek, through bushes of hazelnut, elderberry, and coffeeberry. Cross a wooden bridge and turn left on Bills Trail. Lush foliage thrives beneath the moss-coated trunks of bay laurel trees, and ferns grow along the moist trail. Columbine and forget-me-nots grow among the spring greenery, and in summer and fall, golden grasslands ripple toward the coast on the other side of Devils Gulch.

After 0.8 mile, you veer left on a small path that descends gently into a ravine and reaches the falls in 0.1 mile. Water cascades down step-like rocks in wet months, and ferns and mosses sprout on the moist hillside. Retrace your steps to reach the trailhead.

Barnabe Mountain Loop on Bills and Ridge trails

From the 1466-foot vantage point atop Barnabe Mountain, clear days allow views of Tomales Bay in the north all the way to Mt. Diablo in the south. Shaded, gradual switchbacks comprise the first half of this route; after an abrupt but brief push to the summit, your return route descends steeply to the redwood forest along Lagunitas Creek.

Distance: 9.6 miles, with 6.4-mile option
Type: Loop
Difficulty: Strenuous
Facilities: Toilets, water, picnic tables, and grills at Devils Gulch Horse Camp
Regulations: No dogs. Bikes allowed on fire roads. Horses allowed on fire roads and some trails.
Driving Directions: Continue on Sir Francis Drake Highway for 1 mile beyond the main park entrance and campground to the signed DEVILS GULCH HORSE CAMP on the right side of the road. Park in the gravel pullout on the left.

Begin on the paved road from Sir Francis Drake Highway, high above Devils Gulch Creek, in a forest of bay laurel, big-leaf maple, California buckeye, and alder. Veer right after 0.1 mile on a narrow dirt path, lined by hazelnut, elderberry, coffeeberry, and poison oak. Across a wooden bridge, begin a gradual climb out of the gulch on Bills Trail. Dense tree cover shades lush foliage and moss coats bay laurel trunks. Look for columbine and forget-me-nots in spring.

You pass the turnoff to Stairstep Falls after 0.8 mile and continue up the hillside on long, gentle switchbacks. After crossing a number of wooden bridges, you near the first ridge. The trees begin to thin and grassy slopes extend into the forest cover. Bills Trail ends after 4.0 miles from the trailhead, and you turn left on the Barnabe Trail and make a final steep burst to the summit. Buckeye and bay laurel dot the open slopes, but don't offer shade, and mugwort, cow parsnip, sticky monkeyflower, and wild cucumber line the wide, exposed trail.

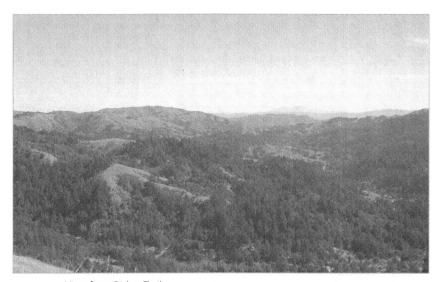

View from Ridge Trail

When you reach the ridgetop after 0.3 mile on the Barnabe Trail, turn left to climb the last few hundred yards to the peak, where you'll have views of Mt. Tamalpais to the southeast, Tomales Bay and the Point Reyes peninsula to the northwest, and volcanic Black Mountain almost directly north.

To return to the trailhead on the longer loop, descend on the Ridge Trail, a wide fire road. Below you, the mountain's slopes fold into forested draws, and residential enclaves in the town of Lagunitas encroach on the open rolling hills. Redwoods cover the hillside across Sir Francis Drake Highway, and the Kent Lake spillway sends water into Lagunitas/Papermill Creek. The Ridge Trail crosses a few stands of Douglas-fir and bay laurel, where thimbleberry and hazelnut line the trail, but the route is mostly exposed until it nears the creekbed and the Riding and Hiking Trail.

You can hear cars on Sir Francis Drake Highway as the trail descends steeply into the creek canyon. In spring, magnificent clarkia—called red ribbons—cover a rocky hillside, accompanied by the bright blossoms of Indian paintbrush. You join the wide, flat Riding and Hiking Trail next to the creek (6.2 miles from the trailhead) and reach Irving Picnic Area after less than a mile. The paved Cross Marin Trail goes straight, on a bridge over Sir Francis Drake Highway, and continues to the main park campground. You veer right on the Riding and Hiking Trail and follow the narrow path beneath bay laurel and oaks. You descend into two gulches, crossing Barnabe Creek at the second, and then meet a fire road where you turn right.

The wide trail makes a short climb and veers left across exposed grassy slopes and through shady pockets of bay laurel. Keep right where a trail heads down toward the road (to Madrone Group Camp). After 1.9 miles from Irving Picnic Area (8.6 miles from the trailhead) you reach the Barnabe Trail. Turn left and descend the wide, rocky trail. You soon cross a stretch of open hillside and re-enter the forest, and then reach the bridge over Devils Gulch Creek and the junction with Bills Trail. Retrace your steps 0.3 mile to Sir Francis Drake Highway.

To take the shorter route back to the trailhead from the peak, retrace your steps on the Barnabe Trail, pass Bills Trail, and continue all the way on the steeply descending Barnabe Trail to the initial junction with Bills Trail, just 0.3 mile from the trailhead. Turn left to reach Sir Francis Drake Highway.

References and
Selected Readings

HISTORY AND NATURAL HISTORY

Alt, David D., and Hyndman, Donald W. *Roadside Geology of Northern California*. Missoula, MT: Mountain Press Publishing Co., 1975.

Bakker, Elna. *An Island Called California*. 2nd ed. Berkeley, CA: University of California Press, 1984.

Evens, Jules C. *The Natural History of the Point Reyes Peninsula*. Point Reyes, CA: Point Reyes National Seashore Association, 1988.

Galloway, Alan J. *Geology of the Point Reyes Peninsula, Marin County, CA*. Sacramento, CA: California Division of Mines and Geology, 1977.

Gilliam, Harold. *Weather of the San Francisco Bay Region*. 2nd ed. Berkeley, CA: University of California Press, 2002.

Hart, John. *Farming on the Edge: Saving Family Farms in Marin County, California*. Berkeley, CA: University of California Press, 1991.

Hill, Mary. *California Landscape: Origin and Evolution*. Berkeley, CA: University of California Press, 1984.

Howell, John Thomas. *Marin Flora: Manual of the Flowering Plants and Ferns of Marin County, California*. Berkeley, CA: University of California Press, 1970.

Livingston, Dewey. *A Good Life: Dairy Farming in the Olema Valley: A History of the Dairy and Beef Ranches of the Olema Valley and Lagunitas Canyon.* San Francisco, CA: National Park Service, Department of the Interior, 1995.

_____ *Ranching on the Point Reyes Peninsula: A History of the Dairy and Beef Ranches Within Point Reyes National Seashore, 1834–1992.* San Francisco, CA: National Park Service, Department of the Interior, 1993.

Mason, Jack. *Point Reyes: The Solemn Land.* 3rd ed. Inverness, CA: North Shore Books, 1980.

_____ *Earthquake Bay: A History of Tomales Bay, California.* 2nd ed. Inverness, CA: North Shore Books, 1980.

GUIDEBOOKS

Martin, Don and Kay. *Point Reyes National Seashore: A Hiking and Nature Guide.* San Anselmo, CA: Martin Press, 1992.

Whitnah, Dorothy. *Point Reyes: A Guide to the Trails, Roads, Beaches, Campgrounds, and Lakes of Point Reyes National Seashore.* 3rd ed. Berkeley, CA: Wilderness Press, 1997. Out of print.

MAPS

Point Reyes National Seashore & Surrounding Area Recreation Map. Berkeley, CA: Wilderness Press.

Point Reyes National Seashore Trail Map. San Rafael, CA: Tom Harrison Maps.

Trails of Northeast Marin County. San Francisco, CA: Pease Press.

WEBSITES

www.npca.org/across_the_nation/park_pulse/point_reyes
www.tomalesbay.net
www.nps.gov/pore

Index

P

MAP INDEX

Also available from **WILDERNESS PRESS**

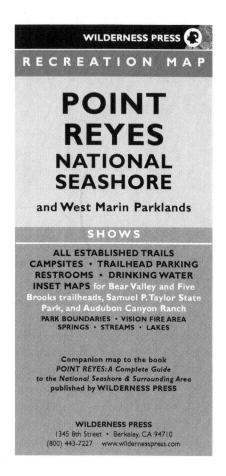

WILDERNESS PRESS

RECREATION MAP

POINT REYES
NATIONAL SEASHORE
and West Marin Parklands

SHOWS

**ALL ESTABLISHED TRAILS
CAMPSITES • TRAILHEAD PARKING
RESTROOMS • DRINKING WATER
INSET MAPS** for Bear Valley and Five
Brooks trailheads, Samuel P. Taylor State
Park, and Audubon Canyon Ranch
PARK BOUNDARIES • VISION FIRE AREA
SPRINGS • STREAMS • LAKES

Companion map to the book
*POINT REYES: A Complete Guide
to the National Seashore & Surrounding Area*
published by WILDERNESS PRESS

WILDERNESS PRESS
1345 8th Street • Berkeley, CA 94710
(800) 443-7227   www.wildernesspress.com

Folding 4-color topographic map shows Point Reyes
National Seashore and vicinity, including Samuel P.
Taylor State Park, Tomales Bay State Park, Audubon
Canyon Ranch Bolinas Lagoon Preserve, parts of
GGNRA, and other West Marin parklands.

26" x 35" unfolded

ISBN 978-0-89997-465-1